Henry Goode Wright

Uterine Disorders : Their Constitutional Influence and Treatment

Henry Goode Wright

Uterine Disorders : Their Constitutional Influence and Treatment

ISBN/EAN: 9783337119898

Printed in Europe, USA, Canada, Australia, Japan

Cover: Foto ©Suzi / pixelio.de

More available books at **www.hansebooks.com**

UTERINE DISORDERS:

THEIR

CONSTITUTIONAL INFLUENCE

AND

TREATMENT.

BY

HENRY G. WRIGHT, M.D., M.R.C.P.

M.R.C.S.L., L.S.A., FELL. MED.-CHIR. SOC., F.R.M.S., &c.

PHYSICIAN TO THE SAMARITAN HOSPITAL FOR DISEASES OF WOMEN.

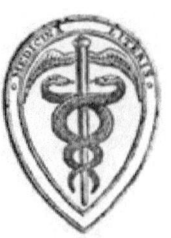

LONDON:
JOHN CHURCHILL & SONS, NEW BURLINGTON STREET.
MDCCCLXVII.

LONDON:
SAVILL, EDWARDS AND CO., PRINTERS, CHANDOS STREET,
COVENT GARDEN.

TO

Thomas Cam, Esq., F.R.C.S.

SURGEON TO THE HEREFORD INFIRMARY,

ONCE MY MASTER, ALWAYS MY FRIEND,

I DEDICATE THIS BOOK,

IN RECOGNITION OF MANY KINDLY SERVICES TO ME AND MINE.

London, 1867.

PREFACE.

There already exist so many comprehensive and trustworthy text-books about Diseases peculiar to Women, that the motives which have induced publication of this work need a few words of explanation.

When required, many years ago, to undertake the charge of a large number of women suffering from uterine disorders, I experienced considerable difficulty in endeavouring to reconcile, for practical use, the discrepant opinions as to the pathology and treatment of such cases. The last books afforded precise information as to the latest views; but a certain disadvantage attended this very exactness,—for that scrupulous impartiality which records with equal favour all opinions, however conflicting, which supplies knowledge and delegates the work of judgment, is rather admirable than practically useful.

As initiative to my personal study of the subject of Diseases of Women, I determined to work through its early history. This long and laborious task afforded certain curious and significant results; some of which are embodied in the introductory chapter. In the subsequent parts of this work I have endeavoured to turn to account the method which I early adopted for my own guidance. There is no disease without some foregone disorder; and the importance of discriminating the causes of disorder in its various stages, led to a recognition of the comparative value of remedies—to adapting the plan of treatment to the exigencies of each case.

It is only after a somewhat exceptional experience, and the study of notes accumulated from thousands of cases, that I venture to speak somewhat authoritatively on certain points yet in dispute, and to suggest various new methods of treatment in uterine disorder and disease. Wherever this responsibility is assumed, it is marked by the use of the personal pronoun, signifying that I hold and defend the position thus adopted.

It is no part of the purpose of this work to discuss discrepancies of opinion. My endeavour has been to build up from sound materials a method of investigation which shall enable the varieties of uterine disorder and disease to be understood, distinguished, and treated according to the ordinary principles of pathology. Elaborate cultivation of one small plot in the field of medical science need not constitute the labourer a specialist, so long as his work is openly and honestly done. I contend that diseases of the womb obey the same laws, and are just as amenable to rational treatment, as diseases of other organs of the body, neither more nor less. Indeed, the peculiarities of the physiological life of the womb render this correlation even more remarkable, and throw still further into the shade those special doctrines concerning uterine pathology—

> "Which had not been if reason ruled,
> Or wisdom wove the web."

H. G. W.

66, HARLEY STREET,
    CAVENDISH SQUARE.

SYNOPSIS.

CHAPTER I.

THE HISTORICAL DISORDER OF UTERINE PATHOLOGY.

Modern revival of uterine pathology; the English and French schools, pp. 1—5. The gynæcology of the Egyptians, of the Israelites, of the Greeks, of the Romans, 5—7. The Alexandrian school, Aëtius, 7—12. The Arabian school, 12—14. The history of the speculum, 14—19. The early European schools, 20—21. Primerose, 21—23. The mischief of modern specialism, 23—25.

CHAPTER II.

DISORDERS OF PLACE.

The order of place, pp. 27—28. The dynamic influences, 28—36. The vascular influences, 36—43. Uterine displacement, 43—48. Prolapsus, active, 49; passive, 52. Treatment, 53. Pessaries, 51, 56. Hydrochlorate of ammonia, 59. Cases, 60. Anteflexion of uterus, 63—67. Anteversion, 67—72. Retroversion, 73. Retroflexion, 74. Treatment, 74—79. Cases, 79—81. Supporting pessaries, 82—84. New intra-uterine spring pessary, 86. Lateral displacement of the uterus, 88—89. Displacement of ovary, 89—91. General treatment of displacements, 91—93. Rest, 93. The bath, 93. Injections, 94. Medicines, 95.

CHAPTER III.

DISORDERS OF FUNCTION.

The natural history of menstruation, pp. 79—112. Amenorrhœa, 112. Emmenagogues, 113. Systemic amenorrhœa, 114. Treatment, 116—118. Ovarian amenorrhœa, 118—121. Uterine amenorrhœa, 121. Use of ergot, 123—125. Suppression of menstruation, 125; of mental origin, 126; of physical origin, 127—132. Joint-pains attending amenorrhœa, 133—136. Vicarious menstruation, 136—140. Menorrhagia, 140—144. Systemic menorrhagia, 144—146. Ovarian menorrhagia, 146—147. Uterine menorrhagia, 147—150. Treatment, 151—157. Dysmenorrhœa, 157. Systemic dysmenorrhœa, 159—166. Ovarian dysmenorrhœa (neuralgic, capsular, and stromal), 167—173. Uterine dysmenorrhœa (neurotic, structural, obstructive, and membranous), 173—188. Leucorrhœa, 188—199. Coincident infra-mammary pain, 200. Treatment, 200—205. Sterility (systemic, ovarian, and uterine), 205—209.

CHAPTER IV.

DISORDERS OF STRUCTURE.

The order of structural change, pp. 210—214. The inflammation theory, 215—221. Cacoplasia, 223—224. Cancer, 224—229. Treatment, 229—232. Epithelioma, 232, 233. Rodent ulcer, 233, 234. Tubercle, 234, 235. Syphilis, 235—237. Heteroplasiæ, 237, 238. Hyperplasiæ, 238—240. Vascular growths, 240—242. Uterine hypertrophy, 242—244. Fibrous tumours and polypus uteri, 244—255. Aplasia, 255. Granular erosion of cervix, 256—258. Treatment, 258—261. Eruptions on cervix uteri, 261—263. Syphilitic aplasia, 263. True ulceration of the cervix, 264, 265.

UTERINE DISORDERS.

CHAPTER I.

THE HISTORICAL DISORDER OF UTERINE PATHOLOGY.

It is now nearly half a century since professional attention was sharply awakened to the inefficiency of the routine practice then generally pursued in Diseases of Women. It was only by a coincidence that the subject came under consideration both in England and France at nearly the same time. Such concurrent investigations (with sometimes even simultaneous but independent discoveries) are by no means rare in the history of science. Thereby is simply signified so general an advancement in knowledge, either general or special, that the same goal presents itself, and the same means are available to many eager observers; all pressing onwards in the same direction.

The works of Sir Charles Clarke and of Dr. Gooch in this country, and of Recamier and Lisfranc in France, may be accepted as those which exercised the most important influence in directing modern attention to the necessity for a more exact study of Diseases of Women. The distinguishing characteristics of the two schools of uterine pathology were just as strongly marked then as they are now. In this country there was, and still is, a tendency to regard uterine affections as intimately associated with, and in the main originally dependent on, some general derangement—to look on the uterine disorder as " a fragment of a constitutional malady." According to the doctrines of the French school, it is the local ailment which is almost exclusively regarded, the constitutional symptoms being attributed to the wide-spread influence exercised by the demonstrated uterine disease. Of this latter view the most zealous exponents were to be found among those energetic practitioners who first introduced into the practice of this country the methods of local investigation and treatment pursued in the French schools. It cannot be doubted that the sudden and enthusiastic advocacy of a very general employment of The Speculum, prominently and persistently declared to be essential for successful treatment, was met by a somewhat injudicious and unreasonable antagonism; the use of a valuable aid to diagnosis and treatment being confounded with its possible abuse by unskilful or unscrupulous persons. Something of this strong opposition might also have been due to the bold proposition so frequently advanced even to this day, that the world was in dense ignorance about uterine diseases until the speculum of Recamier threw light on the subject.

" It was not till of late years," says Sir J. Simpson,[1] " that we had certain means and measures of knowing when inflammation or when ulceration were present." " I have repeatedly

---

[1] Obstetric Memoirs, p. 3.

been asked," writes Dr. Mitchell, "how it happened that our forefathers treated female diseases successfully, as well as the present generation of medical men, without the use of the speculum. To which I would reply, that many went to the grave with the seat of disease undiscovered."[1] Dr. Tilt commences his elaborate work[2] thus: "The dark ages of uterine pathology extend to 1816, when by showing the possibility of an ocular examination of the womb, and urging the frequent necessity of doing so, Recamier enabled his disciples to apply to diseases of that organ the recognised sound principles of general pathology. Those who followed have necessarily derived precision by adding ocular demonstration to the previously known methods of studying diseases of women." So enthusiastic, indeed, were some of the advocates of the use of the instrument that they did not scruple to adopt very exaggerated views. "What opposition," writes Dr. Balbirnie, "did not Harvey's discovery of the circulation of the blood create! He was an innovator. Jenner also was an innovator. The science of auscultation also was opposed in Great Britain; but all these have long achieved their triumph. Doubtless a similar opposition awaits the speculum. We go forth its advocate; we proclaim ourselves the apostle of the speculum; with that instrument we link our fate, and by that we will stand or fall."[3] Such statements may be fairly held to imply a strong belief that

---

[1] Practical Remarks on the Use of the Speculum.
[2] Uterine and Ovarian Inflammation.
[3] Treatise on Organic Diseases of the Womb.

something new had been accomplished, something special to the age, and signifying a great advance in knowledge on account of recent discovery. But the counter arguments employed were just as indiscreet, and the statements often as exaggerated. And this was the more remarkable, since the key-note of the only true and scientific method of investigating uterine diseases had in reality been struck in the admirable works of Clarke and Gooch. It might then have been fairly urged that, according to the method of research of the English school, all constitutional causes producing disorder should be investigated, all the teachings of physiology and general pathology held in mind, and all the extended knowledge of the influence of remedies, and of hygienic medicinal methods laid under contribution, in order to arrive at a correct diagnosis and to insure a good result from treatment. This would have formed the real innovation: for the use of the speculum, and of every one of the newly suggested means and measures of local investigation introduced by the French school, indicated only a revival of the practice pursued in ancient times; when little was known of physiology or pathology, and still less of the *rationale* of treatment. Had this argument been strongly urged and upheld by the very substantial evidence which a little research might have supplied, it is probable that less prominence would have been given to that exclusive use of local means of investigation which chiefly led to uterine disorders first being considered as a speciality. The evil results which have followed are twofold: " Some men regard the local ailment as everything, others almost lose sight of its existence, and it is difficult to say which is the most mischievous."[1] The warm discussions which led men to range themselves into parties might possibly have given place to a method of research more consistent with true scientific advancement, had the curious history of uterine pathology, how it was anciently studied, and why it came to be disregarded, received its due share of attention.

The earliest records of medicine point to the Egyptians as studying the science, even in the most remote periods of their history. A recently translated papyrus[2] contains a treatise on medicine transcribed about the nineteenth dynasty, but believed by learned Egyptologists to have been written in the time of the early Memphitic kings (2600—3500 B.C.), at least a thousand years before the birth of Moses. Now, a study of those parts of the law of Moses wherein special allusions are made to the hygienics of women, and precautions advised concerning them, indicates very clearly that the prudent regulations enjoined (so necessary under the conditions and climate in which the people lived) were founded on observation of the evils arising from neglect. Moses, we are told, was skilled in all the knowledge of the Egyptians; and the rules and observances mentioned were such as would have struck any acute and inquiring stranger living in a land where medical precepts had gradually influenced the domestic habits of the people. That the Egyptians maintained a world-wide medical repute, even down to far later

---

[1] Dr. West: Diseases of Women.   [2] In the Berlin Collection.

times, we have abundant testimony. Homer expressly mentions them as skilled above all men, and directly descended from Apollo.[1] It is beyond doubt that the earliest Greek physicians derived much of their knowledge from Egypt; and if the essays ascribed to Hippocrates—certainly written in his epoch—represent the direction of observation in his time, it is evident that there was then a very advanced knowledge of the Diseases of Women.

The works of Aretæus and Galen strengthen this belief; for it is important to remember that dicta as to diagnosis and treatment of these disorders indicate very long and careful observation, in order to distinguish accidental conditions compatible with health from those symptomatic of disease. In the works attributed to Galen occurs the earliest allusion to the speculum vaginæ as a distinct instrument from the speculum ani; whilst Aretæus describes ulceration of the womb with a precision which leaves little doubt that he also employed the instrument for diagnosis. These authors both studied at Alexandria and practised at Rome. What Athens had been in philosophy and Corinth in arts, Alexandria continued, for several centuries, to be as a centre of medical lore; and even to have studied there was accepted as a qualification to practise. But there gradually arose at Rome an independent school. Celsus, its most distinguished writer, was an exception to the general rule; as he had

---

[1] Ἰητρὸς δὲ ἕκαστος ἐπιστάμενος πέρι πάντων
Ἀνθρώπων· ἦ γὰρ παιήονός εἰσι γενέθλης.
Odyssey, book iv. l. 231.

neither studied at, nor did he love, the Greek schools. Unfortunately, his most important chapter on uterine maladies is, in great part, lost; but we may judge from a passage in his works that, even in his time, diseases of the genital organs were so far a speciality of the Greek school that he could make it a subject of covert sarcasm. In treating of them he says: "Their nomenclature among the Greeks is not only tolerable, but now fully sanctioned by practice, for they are freely employed in almost every volume, work, or treatise of the physicians; but with us Romans these terms are filthy, and never employed by any one who has a proper regard for modesty in language; therefore it is evident that there is no small difficulty in maintaining at the same time a delicacy of expression whilst delivering the precepts of the art." Whether it was jealousy, or a continuance of that same bitter feeling towards the Grecian schools of medicine previously exemplified by Cato[1] and Pliny,[2] it is evident that some other than the alleged motive prompted Celsus to write this sentence; for, being a shrewd practitioner, he must have known that the morality of the Romans—as described in the sixth satire of Juvenal—scarcely required such tender solicitude. Soon after the death of Galen the great medical school of Alexandria was broken up. Its fame had gradually waned, but the well-stored library still remained, enriched by the addition of the manuscripts from Pergamos, another medical school. So vast were the literary treasures that it is reputed 700,000 volumes were destroyed when the

---

[1] Letter to his son Marcus.   [2] Lib. xxiv. cap. viii.

library was burnt by Omar A.D. 642. How many of these works treated on medicine we can only conjecture. Yet we have good grounds for a surmise that there was collected in that grand library all that the gathered experience of generations had left for preservation. Alexandria had been for centuries the centre of medical teaching; and here must have lived and worked those masters of the art to whom the pupils came for instruction. It was their Alma Mater; where else could the manuscripts be so fittingly preserved? And here, about a hundred and fifty years before the final destruction, an industrious compiler laboured, his lifetime through, to condense into practical form the literature of medicine of the period, working among the stores of the great library. His Magnum Opus is still extant, and is, without doubt, the most valuable existing work on ancient medicine, though but little known.

AETIUS lived at Alexandria; and probably practised there, as he makes mention of cases under his own care. But the chief labour of his life must have been the compilation of his book. It was an endeavour, and probably a successful one, to represent the practice then taught and followed in whatever concerns the diagnosis and treatment of disease; omitting, as far as possible, the discussion of theories and allusions to prevalent squabbles about systems. He refers to and gathers from many authorities, but most conscientiously acknowledges all the sources whence his information is drawn; and he condenses with admirable clearness. His work embraces the whole range of medical science as then known. I purpose only alluding to that section in which he treats of Diseases of Women. In addition to its special historical interest, there are some grounds for believing it to be the only authentic and complete treatise on the subject now extant out of all those which were written previous to the time when Aëtius lived ; for Hieronymus Mercurialis attributes the treatises of Hippocrates on the nature and diseases of women to one of his disciples [1]—a view supported by Schultze and others. The chapter in Celsus is imperfect, as also is the history of treatment in Aretæus.[2] The book " de Gynæciis," in Galen, has been held to be fictitious by most editors. Of the works of Soranus, Oribasius, and Rufus, only fragments remain ; whilst other authors to whom Aëtius refers have their names on the roll of the history of medicine, but their works are entirely lost. Such are Philumenes, Archigenes, Pelagrinus, and Asclepiades. This last (from whom Aëtius takes his chapter on healing of ulcers of the womb) is the only one to whom we find any collateral reference, since Cicero speaks of him as his physician and his friend. Lost also is any notice of that first Moschion to whom Pliny attributes a tract " de Pessariis," and of Antyllus, from whom Paul of Ægina derived a chapter on the same subject.

In the sixteenth book of his work Aëtius treats principally of Disorders of Women, devoting to the subject a hundred and twelve chapters, varying in length from a few lines to several such pages as these. Thirty-seven of these chapters treat of pregnancy, of parturition, and of suckling. There

---

[1] Lib. iv. cap. xx.   [2] Lib. ii. cap. xi.

are six chapters on various kinds of ulceration of the womb, three on abscesses, two on displacements, two on obstructed and imperforate uterus, seven on growths occurring in the vagina or uterus, and eighteen chapters on menstruation and its disorders. He has special chapters for hysteria, fibrous tumours, pelvic abscess, hæmatoma, displacements, &c., and devotes one very long chapter to inflammation of different parts of the uterus and its treatment. Only a series of extracts could convey a just estimate of the extent of special knowledge indicated in these descriptions. But so far as concerns the use of the speculum, it is especially worthy of note that he refers again and again to its employment, as a matter of course, in the diagnosis or treatment of ulceration, of tubercula (polypi) in the neck of the uterus, of sessile growths in the same situation, and of calculi and hæmorrhoïds of the womb ; of imperforate uterus, and abscess of the womb. Digital examination is also mentioned as an ordinary means of investigation, " particularly when there is pain denoting ulceration, which is especially liable to happen on the cervix uteri." The treatment he describes includes most of our modern appliances ; in addition to a special description of the use of the speculum. First and most constantly recommended are medicated pessaries, for which he gives upwards of a hundred formulæ.[1] They included not only the rags smeared with ointment, to which pre-

---

[1] " Dr. Simpson first introduced medicated pessaries into use several years ago!" Ed. Med. Journal, June, 1848, p. 886.

vious writers had referred, but also certain preparations compounded and used exactly as they are now-a-days prescribed. The ingredient which forms the basis must be of such kind that it melts at the temperature of the body; it must be so firm that, when cold, it can be neatly introduced; and the relation of these component parts must be varied according to the nature of the conveyed medicaments. In modern practice wax and lard formed, until very recently, the vehicles. The ancient writers used other ingredients, such as beef and deer marrow, goose fat, &c.; and Aëtius describes how, in making suppositories of this kind, the ingredients are to be melted and mingled and allowed to cool before being used.

The use of sponge tents is also very accurately described by Aëtius; how they must be well dried and smeared with unguent, and introduced (with a thread attached) successively until full dilatation is accomplished. In cases where the canal of the cervix has been imperforate, a tin tube is to be inserted in order to maintain the passage, and a speculum subsequently employed, any exuberant granulations being touched with verdigris.[1] The importance of injections, the use of hip-bath, both plain and medicated, the employment of the douche, and application of fumes and vapours by means of a reed introduced into the vagina and connected with a vessel containing the medicated fluid, are all mentioned as ordinarily employed in

---

[1] The employment of a porte caustique had been previously mentioned by Oribasius. Describing the application of caustics, he adds: Uteri autem vesicæque exulcerationes iisdem remediis curantur sed opus est instrumentis quibus intromittantur."

practice. We may fairly infer this; for Aëtius, throughout his work, so carefully refers any special method of practice to the originator, that whenever his description of treatment has no such acknowledgment we may conclude his description to apply to the treatment ordinarily pursued by the most able practitioners of the day.[1]

In his description of the various displacements of the uterus, Aëtius specially mentions the value of rectal examination in retroversion, and how it may aid re-position; and he states, among other suggestions as to treatment, that the correction of lateroversion of the uterus may be effected *specillo et digito*. Here he probably only referred to an ordinary long probe; the recognition of an instrument, specially used as the uterine sound is employed, was of later date.[2]

Before tracing further the history of the speculum, I may allude to a matter naturally suggested when considering what the practice was when Aëtius lived, how thoroughly it fell into desuetude, and has only been revived in comparatively recent times. There was the experience of many centuries, there was the testimony of acknowledged authorities, and there were always suffering women urgently needing help in old times, as at the present time. And if there was any faith in what Aëtius wrote, and in those whom he quotes, why were

---

[1] In the most recent bibliography of writers on uterine diseases (Scanzoni), the work of Aëtius is not mentioned.

[2] Wierus (1657) gives the first accurate description of an instrument exclusively used for uterine exploration.

their teachings disregarded for upwards of a thousand years? It forms a somewhat curious and significant episode in professional history. After the dispersion of the Alexandrian school, the professors of medicine, though scattered, were still received with honour by their Moslem conquerors. What they could teach was eagerly gathered, except when their instruction clashed with any tenet of the Mahommedan creed. The Arabian school, which then arose, comprised equally industrious workers and equally accurate observers. But the study of Diseases of Women was not cultivated among them; for there was an insuperable bar to the attainment of practical experience on the subject. It was against the Mahommedan creed that women, even in their suffering, should undergo personal examination except by one of their own sex. Their degraded social condition prevented their attaining any such position as that to which the women of Greece had vindicated their claims. Even an Hypatia or Agnodice could not have withstood the blighting influence of Moslem sensuality. In the Arabian writings there is only very general mention of Diseases of Women, the matter being principally copied from the Greek books; whilst the local treatment was left in the hands of the midwives. The works of Avicenna, Serapion, and Haly Abbas show how far the Arabian physicians permitted the subject to drop out of notice. It is true that Albucasis, one of the latest writers of the school, refers to these diseases at greater length, but he appears from his writings to have been a Jew. It is he who first mentions herpes of the uterus, and the use of an air pessary for the vagina.[1] Then, as to this day in the East, the midwives undertook the work. One of them, Trotula (thirteenth century), published a treatise on uterine disorders, in which she expressly mentions that many Saracenic women practised at Salerno.

Reverting to the speculum, it is doubtful if the history of any single instrument has been so well preserved. We find it figured in Scultetus, and his description is as follows (the engraving is accurately copied on opposite page): "Fig. 2 is an instrument which they call 'speculum ani et vaginæ uteri,' in that by its help ulcers of the rectum and of the vagina and uterus may be seen, to be carefully observed according to their extent and kind. The part of the speculum, A, drawn open and called male, is applied for men; but the closed part, B, is applied to women, whence it is called female." This is a modification for general purposes, but "Fig. 4 is the large speculum matricis, and is only used for women, when a dead fœtus has to be cut away or an ulceration of the womb to be inspected." To illustrate the method of using this speculum, he gives a representation of a woman with the instrument introduced and dilated; he describes it as that which Paulus Ægineta mentions, whose words he correctly quotes as follows:

"The person using the speculum should measure with a

---

[1] In fracture of the os pubis. He says: "Accipe vesicam ovis et stringe super foramen ejus canulam arundinis et intromitte vesicam totam in vulvam ejus. Deinde suffla in canulam cum virtute donec infletur vesica intra vulvam, fractura enim redit." The process is identical with that recently proposed in cases of mollities ossium.

probe the depth of the woman's vagina, lest the tube of the speculum being too long it should happen that the uterus be pressed upon. . . . . . The tube is to be introduced having

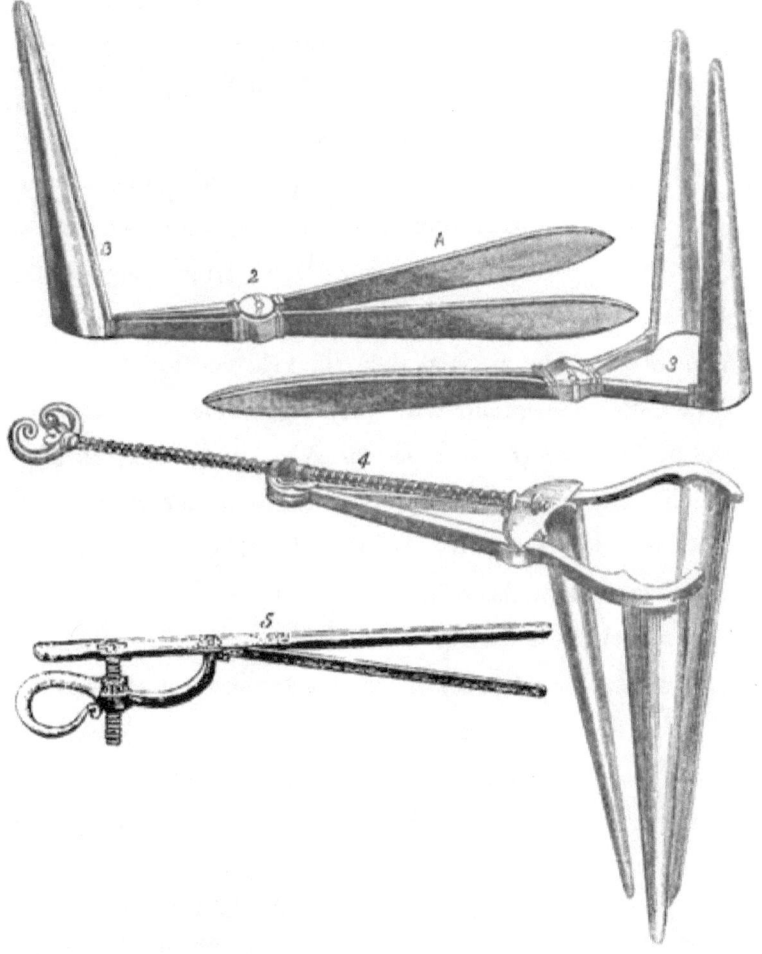

the screw at the upper part, and the speculum is to be held by the operator, but the screw turned by the assistant; so that the laminæ of the tube being separated, the vagina may be dilated."[1]

Now Paul of Ægina lived upwards of a century after the time of Aëtius; and this very description is an almost verbatim copy from that author, but without the conscientious acknowledgment which I have mentioned as characterizing the book of Aëtius, whose description runs thus:

" Per specillum sinus muliebris profunditatem dimetiatur ut ne major dioptræ tibia uterum comprimat . . . . oportet autem tibiam immittere, cochleâ ad supernam partem vergente, et dioptram quidem a chirurgo teneri cochleam vero per ministrum circumverti ut diductis tibiæ plicis sinus distendatur."[2]

The same description, with very slight difference, is to be found in Albucasis (fourteenth century). And it may be conjectured that Scultetus was acquainted with the instrument, but not with its correct use, since in the plate he represents it as introduced with the handle downwards.[3] It is because of this historical reference that I first mention the illustrations of John Schultz (or Scultetus, as he styled himself in the fashion of those days). He was a pupil of Hieronymus Fabricius (1620), who also delineates a three-bladed speculum, whilst others still more complicated are represented by Galbelchouer

---

[1] Lib. vi. cap. lxxiii.   [2] Lib. xvi. cap. lxxxvi.

[3] Armamenta Chirurgica, 1650, engraved from the folio edition. The plates in the smaller copies are very inferior, and frequently altered. The engraving in the original comprises several other uterine instruments, but I have only here represented that marked Fig. 5, on account of its identity in principle with the modern hysterotome.

(1627) and Ambrose Paré (1640). There can be no doubt of the purpose of the speculum as depicted by them; but a still earlier writer, Jacobus Rueffus[1] (1587), has a drawing of a somewhat similar instrument, which he calls the speculum matricis, and describes as employed for dilating the os uteri in difficult parturition, "expedienda instrumenta et præces piæ ad Deum fundendæ." He figures also an apertorium for the same purpose, and the first smooth-bladed obstetric forceps.

From the time of the revival of medicine we find allusions to the use of the speculum becoming more distinct and frequent. In some works it is figured, in many its use for investigating uterine diseases is mentioned as a matter of course. Usually the three-bladed speculum was employed. Wierus (1657) somewhat modified it by making the blades flat; and its frequent use may be inferred from the general description which Garengeot appends to his elaborate representation of it: "L'usage de speculum matricis est de dilater le vagin pour y apercevoir quelques maladies et pour y opérer."[2] A still more complicated instrument is figured by Arnaud in his "Mémoires de Chirurgie" (London, 1798). With this the vagina was dilated by six wires, opening to a considerable extent by a most ingenious mechanical adaptation. Thus there is a tolerably

---

[1] His work, "De Conceptu et Generatione," has a quaint allegorical woodcut representing the Temptation. The tree of knowledge of good and evil has a human skeleton for its stem and trunk, the arms spreading out into fruit-bearing branches with the serpent coiled among them.

[2] Traité des Instrumens de Chirurgie les plus utiles (1727).

continuous history of the speculum from the time of Aëtius down to the present day.

But in the year 1818 there were disinterred at Pompeii

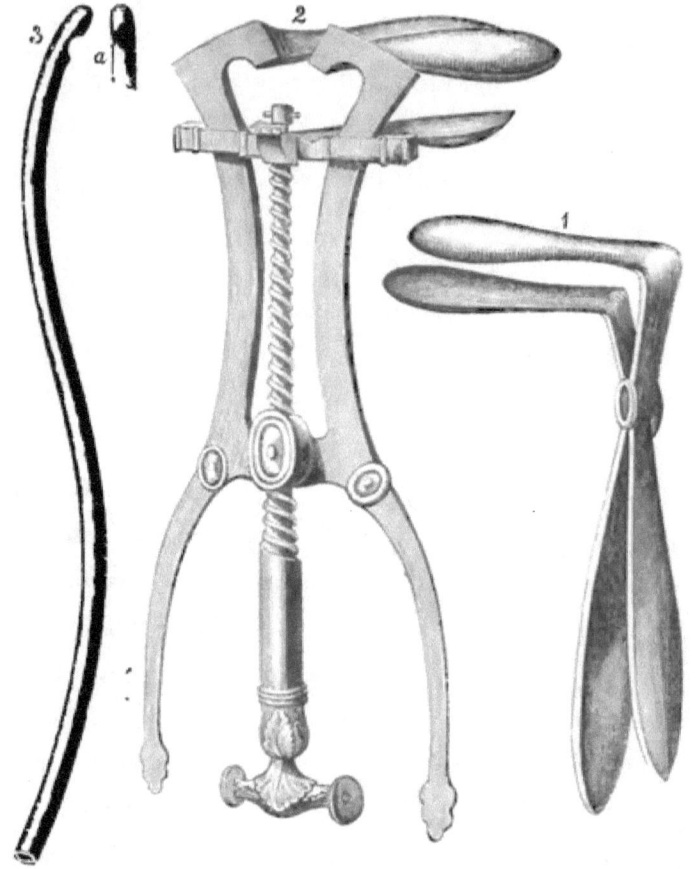

1. The bi-valve speculum.   2. The three-bladed uterine dioptra, the handles folding on hinges for convenience of carriage.   3 is identical in form with the female catheter now most frequently used for relieving the bladder after operations.

a number of surgical instruments, such as were probably in ordinary use when that city was overwhelmed, A.D. 79, four centuries before the time of Aëtius. Among these instruments were two specula, now preserved in the Museo Borbonico, at Naples, and which are here engraved from the officially-authorized works of Dr. C. B. Vulpes.[1]

The learned editor has repeated an error committed by Scultetus, who represented the three-bladed speculum as introduced with the handle downwards, notwithstanding the clear description of Aëtius and Paul of Ægina already quoted. This error was corrected in the quarto edition of Scultetus subsequently published at Paris, where the position of the instrument is correctly delineated. There can be no doubt that these specula or dioptra were such as Aëtius referred to; with probably such improvements as we might suppose to have been suggested in the centuries intervening between the date of the destruction of Pompeii and his era.

I have dwelt at some length on the history of the speculum, since there exists a general belief among the profession—how engendered and fostered it is needless to inquire—that the employment of local remedies and the use of the speculum for elucidation of uterine diseases is quite a triumph of modern special research. But if we are content to credit the practitioners of past times with an unexpected amount of knowledge about uterine diseases and their local treatment, it must not be forgotten that their writings are sadly deficient in another

---

[1] Illustrazione di tutti gli instrumenti chirurgici scavati in Ercolano e in Pompei e che ora conservansi nel Real Museo Borbonico di Napoli. Dal Car. Benedetto Vulpes. 1847.

and perhaps even more important direction. I allude to the constitutional treatment of uterine disorders, and especially to those correlative influences which so frequently determine the local malady. In all such cases exclusive local treatment can afford but temporary relief; and this is neither a satisfactory nor a scientific result. But even to disentangle all the ravelled threads of inter-causation and accurately weigh the value of every symptom would avail us little, if we had not the means of combating successfully the recognised morbid conditions. Without the aid afforded by chemistry in providing us with remedies, our most elaborate pathological researches would only illustrate the shrewd observation which Asclepiades made in reference to the Hippocratic doctrine, that it was " a meditation on death."

The Arabian physicians laboured in the laboratory and laid the foundations of that great science which has supplied so many valuable remedies for the cure of disease. Alchemy was the plaything of Chemistry's childhood—but the time spent in its pursuit was not all wasted. They sought the Elixir of Life to cure disease and renovate decay; believing that the discovery of the philosopher's stone would reveal this also. The first principles of physiology and of commercial exchange were ignored by men who aspired to absolute immortality and boundless wealth; just as the search for an universal solvent was prosecuted without ever considering what should contain it when discovered.

In the writings of the early European physicians on uterine disorders the influence of the Arabian school is clearly traceable.

They allude but vaguely to causation or to local treatment; but the use of empirical remedies, and of an uncouth polypharmacy, especially marks the period. Thus, for example, Rueffus advises for the cure of sterility a mixture containing thirty-eight ingredients, and a bath comprising thirty-three. The great reaction which occurred at the time of the revival of European literature was especially notable for the publication of many works on uterine diseases. It was not enough that Wolphius should gather into a single work various short treatises on the subject, chiefly by ancient authors, but the book was in such demand that Schenckius and Spatius subsequently produced similar reprints. In addition to those works of reference and to the editions of classic authors by Aldus and other publishers, there appeared in the seventeenth and eighteenth centuries a number of books, more or less original, treating exclusively of Diseases of Women. From these I select one as representing the available knowledge of the period, and illustrating my opinion as to the importance and originality of the views on uterine pathology advocated by the English school. The work to which I refer is, I believe, the earliest treatise on Diseases of Women by a graduate and practitioner of this country—as it is certainly the most complete, sensible, and practical of all the works on the subject published at that time.

JACOBUS PRIMEROSE was a Scotchman by extraction, studied in Paris, graduated at Oxford, and practised at Hull. His work, "De Morbis Mulierum," was published at Rotterdam, and bears the date of 1665. He was evidently a man of decided opinions and original thought, with a thorough knowledge of classical professional literature. Hippocrates, Galen, and Aëtius are his principal authorities, though he alludes to the opinions of modern authors, and does not scruple to condemn, in no measured terms, those whose views do not square with his own. His book includes sixty-one chapters, giving evidence throughout of keen and original observation. He mentions the use of the speculum, as a matter of course, wherever the condition of the cervix uteri has to be investigated. Other appliances, pessaries, injections (both vaginal and intra-uterine), fumigations, medicated poultices, plasters, and instruments, receive due notice. But the distinguishing characteristic of the book of Primerose is the careful attention paid to those points of treatment which were most disregarded by the writers of his time. The air to be breathed, the food to be eaten, the clothing to be worn, and the baths to be used, are indicated with peculiar care, the natural mineral waters being advised in appropriate cases. The third book is chiefly devoted to the general influence of uterine disorders; taking notes of cases of epilepsy, of affections of the heart, the spleen, the liver, the stomach, and the head, depending on uterine disease, and describing uterine pains which occur independent of any local disease. The mental influences originating from depraved uterine action are dwelt on at length in a chapter on melancholia. Hysteria, its history and diagnosis, is described with a practical shrewdness and accuracy which acquires especial interest from a comparison with the well-known and contemporary contribution of Sydenham on the subject. Primerose wrote from a mind largely stored with the lore of those who had studied uterine pathology. His hysteria was that which took its derivation from ὑστέρα—the womb. Sydenham wrote as a general observer of the phenomena of disease; and the notable errors of each are to be traced to the point of view from which the subject was exclusively regarded.[1] That the work of Primerose has lain unnoticed for two centuries is probably owing to the circumstance that he, being, as I have said, an opinionated man, committed himself by a vehement opposition to the doctrines about the circulation of the blood which Harvey introduced into this country.

It is scarcely necessary to point out that a recognised speciality in medicine, only thus segregated because its results are attributed to modern research and discovery, has its foundations seriously disturbed so soon as we recognise that the greater part of the claims to originality can be proved untenable. Much additional corroborative evidence might be readily adduced: but

---

[1] Whilst investigating the special literature of this subject, I had occasion to refer to a pedantic "Encyclopædia Medicinæ," by J. Dolæus, 1684, which contains a book on uterine diseases. It has some prefatorial laudatory lines by Sydenham, not mentioned in the biographies of the father of English medicine, commencing thus:—

> "Sic documenta damus doctrinæ sacra probatæ
> Quid valeant humeri judicet ut sapiens
> Gratulor ex animo Deus isthæc cœpta secundet
> Sit nomen magnum clare Dolæe tuum
> Cum voto exoptatissimæ felicitatis scripsit.

"Londini, 1683."   "Thom. Sydenham, M.D.

my present purpose will be sufficiently served if any of the time and talent now being wasted in exploring an already overworked mine be diverted to more worthy investigations and more healthy methods of research. I fully believe that if English practitioners had followed the teachings of their own school, and availed themselves judiciously of the knowledge garnered by generations of observant men, we should have been spared many unseemly professional discussions, the enunciation of certain preposterous theories, and denunciations which assuredly prove that either the accuser or the accused must be very much in the wrong. It is by the exclusive focussing of professional attention to one point, which hence acquires an exaggerated importance, that the great character of Medicine as a cumulative science is distorted in its development, and that special branches of it become warped in the growth. This is especially true as regards modern uterine pathology. The eccentric theories of early times were not refuted, since there existed no facilities for professional discussion or controversy. But the same difficulties also prevented their wide publication; so that we have now, probably, a more exact knowledge of the different views held by ancient authors of the Greek and Roman schools, than was possessed by the most learned contemporary physicians. If many of the theories then propounded now appear preposterous and absurd, it is at least certain that the authors were earnest in what they wrote. Their errors were rather due to deficiency of knowledge than to want of judgment. The time had not yet arrived, when attention could be arrested by the constantly crying out of one thing, and crying that one thing very loud.

In early times there was no wide dissension as to the pathology of uterine disorders; to the great comfort of the learners, who knew what to believe; for the number of those content to think for themselves, who pin their faith to no man's sleeve, was then and is now comparatively small. The student of modern uterine pathology, if he accept every direction written for his observance, and be guided in his practice by the latest propounded views, will assuredly be worse off than the men of old, who acknowledged their ignorance, trusted very much to nature, and were content to leave bad alone, lest bad should be made worse; for the clash of modern theories about uterine disorders, and the bitter controversies that followed, has rather tended to confuse than to guide. It is only by long practical experience and close observation that some explanation of these diversities of opinion is gathered; where cases constantly come under notice which *might* be so read off as to illustrate the views of special theorists, and therefore to justify any method of treatment which a prepossessed observer would consider applicable. It would be a labour equally tedious and unprofitable to record at length the modern opinions on uterine pathology which have been propounded, refuted, and again advanced since attention was reawakened to this subject. I have attentively read what has been written, and it appears to me undoubtedly true that the strongest assertions are throughout on the weakest side—that those nearest to the truth have confided in it most, believing that it was great and would prevail.

CHAPTER II.

DISORDERS OF PLACE.

THE ORDER OF PLACE.—The ovaries, the uterus and its appendages, the vagina with the parts which sentinel its entrance, constituting the Female Generative Cycle, have, in common, numerous provisions which regulate their action in health, and exercise an important influence under conditions of local disorder or disease. Precise knowledge of the structural anatomy of all these parts is an essential preliminary to the study of their co-ordinate action; but the recognition of their inter-relations is equally important for unravelling the tangled threads of causation, and determining the meaning of symptoms.

Considering the ovaries and uterus, as seen in place, there is no reasoning, inductive or analogical, by which any relation between them could be predicated; for the ovary is a ductless gland, and the tubes of Fallopius appear to open into the cavity of the peritoneum. But when the functions of these organs are considered, it is impossible to misconstrue the relation between the physiological duties assigned to the different parts which form the female generative cycle.

Co-ordination of place as well as of action is essential to the due performance of the various duties which the uterus and its ancillary organs have to fulfil. When considering the order and disorder of place, the chief place may be thus conceded to the uterus; when fulfilment of function comes to be investigated, the ovaries will assume the primary importance.

The finite purpose of the organs which make up the female generative cycle, requires a sequent transference of the ovum, the germ, and the fœtus from ovary to uterus, from uterus to external life; and this transference implies an existing order of place between the organs themselves. The maintenance of this order is equally important under all conditions which involve exercise of the uterine functions. Displacements always induce suffering; they prevent or arrest gestation, or render it abnormal; and they very frequently determine the conditions under which disorder passes into disease.

Some mention of the provisions made for insuring an order of place may here precede consideration of its disorders; since the success of the treatment to be pursued must, in every case, materially depend on prior recognition of the various ways in which the healthy conditions may have been disarranged.

Two co-ordinate physical influences exercise an important power in determining the position of the uterus. These are—

1. The dynamic } arrangements.
2. The vascular

1. *The Dynamic Arrangements.*—In the adult virgin, the uterus and ovaries, weighing together about 13 drachms, appear

to be slung between the folds of the broad ligament, and thus sustained. This relation was long considered to afford a sufficient explanation of the mechanism by which these organs are retained in place, and enabled to yield, on occasion, to the influences exercised by neighbouring parts. Certain later observers dissented from this decision, and accredited the vagina as the chief agent in maintaining the uterus in its position. The opinions expressed on either side are very decided. Dr. Matthews Duncan[1] upholds the statement of John Bell, that "the firmness and structure of the vagina support the womb;" and says of the broad ligaments, "these so-called ligaments have neither the structure nor function of parts ordinarily so named."

Dr. D. Davies,[2] agreeing with Morgagni, thus states his views when describing the broad ligaments of the uterus:—"It is not true that the broad ligaments are so totally devoid of claim, as has been lately very generally represented, to the designation of ligaments. If, indeed, ligaments be cords or bands, of whatever structure, used for fastening parts to parts, there are certain portions of the tissues in question true ligaments."

The strong points of the rival arguments are, on the one hand, that a specially dilatable tube like the vagina can of itself have no adequate supporting power, resembling (as it has been aptly put) 'a cup and ball, without the solidity and natural power of resistance of the cup.' On the other side it is urged

---

[1] Edinburgh Medical and Surgical Journal, 1854.
[2] Obstetric Medicine, vol. i. p. 220.

that a duplication of delicate serous membrane like the broad ligament is unfitted to sustain an uterus of the size that the organ often attains in multiparæ; even if no mention were made of the increase in volume and weight which occurs at each pregnancy.

Allowing the validity of both these objections, setting altogether aside the vagina and broad dissepiment of peritoneum as exercising no individual sustentative influences, there yet remains a full and sufficient explanation of the method by which the organs are retained in place, and one which goes far to explain and reconcile the discrepant opinions already cited.

The researches of M. Jarjavay,[1] and the later dissections of Dr. Priestley,[2] on the fasciæ of the female pelvis, have given greater significance to the intimately interlaced connective threads which exist so abundantly in the interspaces of the female pelvis, surrounding and supporting its contained organs in health, and serving to guide or impede the advance of pelvic abscess or of hæmatocele.

Some of the most closely aggregated of these had been previously demonstrated and described as true ligaments, whilst the more generally diffused connective threads were summarily disposed of under the designation of "loose cellular tissue," serving to fill up interspaces and fossa. In truth, all these structures, whether called fasciæ, ligaments, or cellular tissue,

---

[1] Archives Générales de Médecine, 1849.
[2] On Pelvic Abscess and the Fascia of the Pelvis in the Female.—Monthly Journal of Medical Science, 1854.

wherever they exist, fulfil the same office, and are merely modifications of the same material to subserve special exigencies. Throughout the body they are identical in action, in structure, and in chemical composition, exercising a mechanical rather than a vital influence. In the female pelvis the component parts are adjusted to the required sustentative power, varying in closeness of relation, from the internexation constituting fascia, to such an open distribution that the epithet " loose cellular tissue" has been considered sufficiently descriptive.

Speaking with precision, such a definition is obviously incorrect; for the structure thus described is neither loose, nor cellular, nor tissue; which latter word is derived from the Saxon pepan, "to weave," and implies the presence of cross threads, the woof of the warp. The word " loose " has probably been applied because of the ease with which the filaments break down under the finger or scalpel. But this is no standard of their united strength, any more than the individual threads which compose a spider's web represent their conjoint power. So, also, the absolute strength of a rope is far in excess of what could be predicated from separately testing its component threads. In the rope each strand operates at a mechanical disadvantage, having to raise a mass by attachment to one point of it. In the spider's web the fly may be caught at any part, and the symmetry of power which governs the web be thus destroyed; but in the female pelvis the connective fibrillæ, every thread having a distinct purpose and connexions, exercise a sustentative influence, which depends for its perfection on their combined strength. The rope and the spider's web illustrate the influences exercised by ligament and fascia, by fibrous structure or "loose cellular tissue," whether distributed around the vagina for its support, condensed in the superior pelvic fascia, or spread out between the layers of the broad ligament, the peritoneum of which is thickened, as it is throughout the pelvic cavity, by a reinforcement of strong fibrous tissue.

Thus it is that the vagina exercises an important influence in supporting the womb, though itself destitute of sustentative power; for it is borne up on every side by supporting filaments, which find their common point of attachment in its fibrous sheath, those laterally attached having the most elastic power. This areolar sheath, moreover, exercises a constricting influence; so that the vagina, when at rest, becomes a curved column of firm tissue, flattened from before backwards. Its cavity may be fully dilated with no other result than that of directly shortening each of the connective threads around it. But any movement, upwards or downwards, throws a strain on these elements of support, and takes them at a mechanical disadvantage. Such a departure from the order of place must ensue where a weighty uterus overcomes the sustaining power that the vagina obtains by extrinsic support. But the distress thus caused, and the inordinate strain produced, are very rarely accompanied by any evidence of active protest such as we find where the more highly-vitalized structures of the body are subjected to undue exercise, and tried beyond their endurance. Inflammation of the cellular tissue of the pelvis rarely occurs as a direct consequence of displacement. Throughout the whole body, wherever it is distributed, areolar or 'cellular' tissue exercises a dynamic influence; its immense strength depending everywhere on the combined action of a number of minute elastic threads, apportioned according to the sustentative power required. It allows a certain amount of free motion—varying in each situation, and constituting one of its most important attributes—whether condensed into the form of tendon and ligament, or distributed as a thin layer, such as exists beneath the skin of the body and the muscles of the scalp. Displacement of the uterine organs represents a condition in which the special provisions for affording support, and yet ensuring mobility, are unduly strained in some particular direction. Considering the uterus only, the connective tissue distributed above, on either side, and below the organ,—whether acting directly, as in the folds of the broad ligament and the fibres of the round ligament, or mediately, by attachment to the vagina,—allows a very considerable range of movement, which is perfectly compatible with health. The full bladder, the inflated intestine, or loaded rectum, the descent of the diaphragm during inspiration, and many other causes, induce recurring changes of place. The organ deviates from and recovers its position by the elasticity of that system of supporting agencies now under consideration. The influence they exercise, both by reason of structure and distribution, is eminently antagonistic to jerk. Were the uterus fixed in the pelvis, the least jar of the frame, as in sitting down or when riding, would arrest gestation just as surely as the leap of the stag would shatter its whole frame, had not its parts been so fashioned as to antagonize the violence of the shock. These slight deviations of place in the uterus, constantly occurring, and unfelt by the individual, are best observed where it becomes necessary to employ an intra-uterine sound for diagnosis, when the handle may be seen to move with each descent of the diaphragm on inspiration.

But, in addition to the important purpose already mentioned, a certain physiological value attaches to this recurring variation of place in the uterus and its neighbouring parts. The stimulus of action induces reparation of tissue in all the countless threads of connective structure which, in turn, are exercised by these movements; and this is a necessity where the blood supply is so comparatively sparse. The evil result that would follow inaction is daily seen in the stiffening of the ligaments of unused joints. And the principle is the same throughout; for, compared with highly-organized structures, as those of the lungs or kidneys, the "cellular tissue" is comparatively bloodless. If thereby rendered less liable to inflammation, it has less power of resisting its progress or removing its results. Hence the intractability of pelvic cellulitis. That this serious result rarely happens, in even the most exaggerated cases of uterine displacement, may be explained by what has been already noted; for there is no boundary line between the natural mobility specially provided for and essential to health, and those lesser conditions of displacement which only represent exaggeration in some particular direction of these movements; nor can any distinction be drawn between the latter cases and those of extreme deviation.

At various angles with the fibres of connective tissue, whether acting singly or condensed into fasciæ, there are arranged certain more distinct provisions for equalizing the action or affording additional means of support. The most important of these is the dissepiment of firm fascia, forming a floor to the cavity of the true pelvis, sufficiently strong to support such of the abdominal viscera as may occasionally rest upon it, and firm enough to retain *in situ* the pelvic organs which perforate it. A process of this superior pelvic fascia, so elaborately demonstrated by Dr. Priestley, exercises a more immediate supporting influence on the vagina and uterus. It "takes its origin from the upper border of the thyroid foramen and brim of the true pelvis; descends vertically and slightly inwards;" then "follows a new direction until it reaches the side of the vagina and the most inferior part of the bladder. Here it joins the fibrous sheath enclosing the vagina and neck of the bladder, and with it expands itself upwards as a cellular layer on the fundus of the bladder and neck of the uterus."

That distributed dynamic power which has for its office the maintenance of the order of place in the organs that constitute the generative cycle, is arranged with due regard to some opposing force; or, in other words, to the weight which has thus to be sustained. Any increase of this weight, whether of the womb or its appendages, necessarily, therefore, produces derangement of this order; unless there be provided some corresponding increase of support. Any such absolute increment in weight of the uterus or ovaries must be due to the agency of the blood supply.

2. *The Vascular Arrangements* in the generative cycle of the female represent the highest application of those subtle general adaptations by which the blood is distributed according to local exigencies. For the due supply of the various requirements of different parts of the body there is a special arrangement of the mechanism of the vascular system. This may, perhaps, be most forcibly illustrated by contrast. In the brain the method of the vascular disposition is exactly the opposite of that which obtains in the generative circle. The arterial supply is carefully steadied and guarded. The curved bony canals through which the vessels enter the brain, and those free intercommunications provided by the circle of Willis, are all arranged with such purpose; whilst the large straight veins inserted between dense tissue, so that their action may not be interfered with, indicate how carefully both entrance and exit are guarded, in order to insure an unimpeded and equable flow. The active brain withdraws from the passing blood only a few out of many elements; but

this nutritive eclecticism renders a continuous flow essential to the vitality of the organ; whilst any retardation of venous efflux, any such approach towards stagnation as congestion implies, is inimical to healthy action.

The vascular arrangements of the pelvic organs present an arrangement almost the reverse of that above described. The fully-developed fœtus requires from the blood every element with which it is freighted, and the arterial supply is profuse; but, beyond the capillaries, the current passes slowly onward, filling the tangled plexus and the spongy uterus, and that supplementary provision for retarding the flow which the placenta presents. The venous plexus, obviously a provision for slackening the force and rapid flow of the blood through the adjacent parts, finds its most marked illustration in the pelvic system of the female. The reticulated masses of veins, forming respectively the ovarian, uterine, vaginal and vulvar plexus, well described by Monsieur Roujet, and admirably demonstrated by Mr. J. Reeves Traer, derive their chief interest from their special adaptation to the requirements of the parts,—exercising a double influence. In pregnancy they retard the through current of the blood, enabling a more thorough appropriation of its nutritive elements. But they subserve more direct mechanical purposes in accordance with the requirements of the parts where they exist; and which the usual definition of erectile action very inefficiently explains. Such venous turgescence exercises an important influence over all those conditions which accompany the beginning and end of uterine life. And the maintenance of order, both of place and function, during the period of active uterine life, depends for its integrity very much on the due co-ordination of the vascular arrangements.

The vessels of the ovary freely communicate with those of the uterus, and may be injected from either organ. But the full distension of the ovarian venous plexus exercises a fluid pressure, which, in an organ so situated, must influence its position. It has been conjectured, that this mechanism assists its approximation towards the pavilion of the oviduct. It is by vascular turgescence that the fimbriæ of the Fallopian tubes so distend as to grasp the presenting surface of the ovary, and that the expansion of the pavilion, and the widening of the narrow canal of the oviduct, are determined. Although it may appear that a communication exists between the uterus and abdominal cavity, this is never really the case under ordinary conditions of health. For no effective passage along the Fallopian tube exists, except when the fimbriated extremity is closed by the presenting part of the ovary. This action of the Fallopian tubes is determined from the uterus, whence it receives its supply of blood, only a very minute arterial twig passing to the ovary through the ovario-tubal ligament. The importance of this arrangement is obvious, since the stimulus to action is conveyed from the direction of the uterus.

The large uterine venous plexûs lying on either side of the organ, and communicating freely with the ovarian plexûs above, fulfil a very important office in retarding the progress of the current of blood, as already mentioned. The plexûs of veins around the vagina, and those at the vulvar orifice, exercise a coarctive influence on the passage; they freely communicate with one another, as also with the uterine plexûs, thus completing the venous chain from ovary to the external orifice. There "the veins which collect the blood from the labia, constrictor muscles and mucous membrane of the vagina, and from the erectile tissue forming the vaginal bulb, unite to form a considerable plexus, especially around the vulvar orifice, termed the vaginal plexus. From this plexus branches pass to the vesical, hæmorrhoidal and uterine plexus." (Farre.) "There is this peculiar to the veins, that they communicate with the hæmorrhoidals, and consequently with the venæ portæ." (Winslow's Anatomy.) "The hæmorrhoidal branches inosculate with branches of the internal iliac vein, and thus establish a communication between the portal and general venous system." (Wilson's Anatomist's Vademecum.) This communication demands special notice, as bearing importantly on the subject of uterine displacements.

The condition of the vascular arrangements in health must not be accepted as always representing what takes place in disorder or disease. Thus, the minute vessels of the conjunctiva, which strain off from the blood only such parts as are necessary for nutrition, admit corpuscles so soon as their healthy action is impaired, either by the exercise of excessive impulse, or by relaxation affecting the calibre of the vessels themselves. For the latter condition there needs no exaggeration of vascular impetus; since the mischief evidently depends on deficiency of the resistant power. Such an atonic state may obtain throughout the system in persons of relaxed and enfeebled habit where the sustentative power of the connective tissue is wanting in efficiency. There is little of that firm and well-braced elasticity which accompanies health, and this condition is well expressed by the vernacular term "flabby." In women thus enfeebled, it might be expected, from the peculiar structure of the portal and intra-pelvic veins and plexus, all of them destitute of valves, and for the most part situated among open areolar structures, that even a comparatively small venous communication would enlarge under the pressure of blood seeking exit; especially if its normal course were obstructed. The tortuous course which has to be traversed through the chain of uterine venous plexûs above described, might yet offer a means of transit in cases of congestion of the liver, more free than the portal vein presents; the plexus, along this new route, allowing room by their engorgement for a portion of this diverted current, without immediately interfering with the organs of the female pelvis. There would thus be produced a condition of venous congestion of the chain of plexus, which only differs from that attending menstruation or pregnancy, in the fact that such a mechanical encroachment from the hæmorrhoidal veins follows on a disordered action, and is not determined by a specific vital stimulus, such as induces the catamenial congestion and the vascular arrangements which minister to gestation. Thus, the same conditions which in health serve to readily unload the uterine vessels and prevent congestion, may, if the whole series of plexus be engorged through portal obstruction, induce the very evil they were arranged to prevent. But, it may be urged, the uterus is itself in a spongy state during pregnancy; and at that time can exercise little propulsive force to empty the large and numerous veins which exist throughout its structure. The researches of Kölliker have, however, shown, that as these venous channels increase in size during pregnancy, their middle coat, which before consisted of cellular structure, begins to develop actual muscular fibres.

The relations between hepatic (or portal) obstruction and uterine disorder is a matter of every-day observation, and is conceded by all who have studied the subject. Sir J. Y. Simpson says the biliary and catamenial secretions seem almost vicarious of each other, and observes, "in some cases the cure of an uterine disorder seems almost to rectify the co-existent, and, perhaps, resultant hepatic derangement; while no doubt also in other cases we find ourselves unable to amend or correct uterine diseases and discharges till we have, in the first instance, used appropriate means to modify and correct the attendant hepatic disorder." Sir Charles Clarke had previously noted the connexion between uterine and vaginal flux and some unhealthy state of the liver; especially remarking that the conditions indicative of uterine disorder increased as the hepatic derangements became more marked. A special treatise on this subject was published by Dr. Butler Lane;[1] and Dr.

---

[1] On Functional Diseases of the Liver associated with Uterine Derangements. 1848.

Beauchene,[1] recognising the influence so admirably epitomized by Sir J. Y. Simpson, suggested that acrid bile retained in the blood irritated the uterine nervous system, perverted its vitality, and influenced the periodic flow.

Whatever the theories which have been held in reference to this relation between the portal and uterine circulation, its practical importance has not been disregarded. The application of leeches to the verge of the anus, as a means of relieving congestion of the uterine system, owes its origin to recognition of this important vascular co-ordination. The practice is of considerable antiquity, and supplies one of the very few examples where the ancient method of attending to effects and neglecting causes still prevails. The earliest direct mention is in Hieronymus Capivacceus,[2] who says: "It is important to recognise whether it be advisable to apply leeches to hæmorrhoids. The application of leeches to hæmorrhoids is a method of derivative remedy—that is, of evacuating the blood which settles around the uterine region." Primerose,[3] to whose writings reference has been already made, advances still more decided opinions as to the venous correlations existing between the portal and uterine nervous systems. "The spleen and liver also act in consent with the uterus. For whereas the uterus has many veins, and these specially large, the blood, if checked and vitiated, regurgitates to the liver, whence various

---

[1] Les Maladies Nerveuses des Femmes, p. 108.
[2] Pract: lib. 4, (1617).
[3] De Morbis Mulierum, 1685, lib. 3, cap. 12.

issues of disease, according to the nature of the peccant humour." Almost identical is the remark of Dr. Evory Kennedy, that "an engorged state of the uterus is very liable to alternate with, translate to or co-exist with, congestion of the liver and spleen."

Stahl, whose eccentric theories led to the neglect of much that is valuable in his writings, pointed out with great precision the importance of the vascular co-relation under consideration in his treatise, "De Mensium Insolitis Viis." He says:— "The vessels from the internal iliacs, and the hypogastric ramifications of them, are distributed to the body of the uterus itself, but from the hæmorrhoidal branch to the neck of the organ. This distribution is to be carefully considered, which draws blood through the hæmorrhoidal branch from the vena porta, for the purpose of the menstrual secretion ; and so much the more as it happens that it has hitherto been lightly estimated in relation to our subject."

If the important influences exercised by these dynamic and vascular arrangements, on which the order of position of the uterine organs so much depends, have been described with sufficient clearness, it must be evident that the recognition of displacement should in practice be only initiative to the consideration of its causes, and that the treatment must be fashioned in accordance with the knowledge thus acquired.

THE DISORDERS OF PLACE.—In a very large majority of the cases of uterine displacement this effect has been slowly produced, and the symptoms have gradually increased in intensity. Instances of sudden and forcible displacement, whether flexion, prolapsus, or inversion, approach more nearly to a true dislocation in the suddenness of the attack, and the direct mechanical violence to which the mischief is clearly attributable. Here reposition affords immediate relief, and rest completes the cure, just as in dislocation of a joint. But the cases of Uterine Disorder of Place which most frequently come under notice present a very different history. They vary in extent and direction, so as to defy exact classification. Thus the organ may be fairly bent on itself, may be bodily displaced upwards or downwards, or may be removed from its normal position by mere increase of its natural curve, or by this curve assuming a new and unnatural direction. And so far may these conditions vary and mingle, that the classifications hitherto adopted have been rather for purposes of general description than as absolutely marking the exact displacement in each individual case. Some authors have attempted a more elaborate definition; thus M. Nonat tabulates thirty-nine different deviations of place, compounded out of the three forms of displacement chiefly recognised—prolapsus, version, and flexion of the uterus.

The uterus is tethered in the pelvis; having a considerable range of movement in every direction. The only approach to fixation is an attachment of its lower part to the bladder, this connexion being continuous with a similar attachment of the upper part of the vagina, so that in health the orifice of the cervix uteri maintains a direction corresponding to that of the centre of the distended vaginal canal. This is obviously adapted to ensure insemination. The positional relations of the bladder to the uterus exercise also a further influence. The roomy pelvis of the unimpregnated woman allows the bladder to distend to an enormous extent; and habitual control up to the very extreme that can be borne (a custom not unfrequent with women), tends to increase the vesical capacity. The female bladder is emptied with great rapidity, and the recurrence of these conditions of extreme distension and sudden collapse necessarily implies an inordinate variation in the position of the uterus also, which has a certain importance in the treatment of its disorders of place. Equally mechanical in action is the influence, produced by distension of the rectum with scybalæ; for the gut has been found enlarged to the diameter of a tumbler by this cause, displacing the uterus by the pressure. The position of the uterus changes with each deep inspiration; and where the play of the ribs is restricted, the organ habitually occupies an unusually low position in the pelvis. With tight stays, having stout busks of wood or iron, such as working women wear, the diaphragm has to afford the room required for entrance of air into the lungs. But the movements of abdominal respiration in such cases are chiefly referred to the hypogastriæ parietes, since the weight of the manifold lower garments (which are supported by ligatures at the waist) serves to constrict the very part which in men most responds to the influence exercised by the descent of the diaphragm on deep inspiration. By the uterine sound this variation in place is readily recognised; and the range of movement differs according to the conditions of the examination, whether the patient be loosely clad or compressed by stays. Working women wear these from a mistaken notion that they afford support—not from mere vanity; and under the same erroneous opinion have strong wooden busks, like flat rulers, let into the front of the garment. I have seen deep dents in the sternum and depressions in the linea alba produced by constant pressure of the ends of those abominable things; and I think I must have, in hospital practice, ordered the removal of enough wooden ones to build a boat. The elastic support afforded by the abdominal walls antagonizes the descent of the diaphragm only so long as the healthy condition of them is maintained. But in multiparæ, and in women with large and pendulous bellies, the sustaining power of the parietes is slight. This is well seen in cases of ovariotomy, where the contraction of the abdominal walls on either side the incision varies remarkably. I have known the parietes as lax as damp leather, and in other cases have felt the recti abdominis tensely draw together the internal edges of the incision after extraction of the tumour.

There is also another condition, which, though rarely met with, may be admitted as sometimes modifying the mechanical agency of the abdominal parietes. I have notes of fifteen cases of its occurrence, but have not met with any statistical account as to its frequency. In all of these there was a depressed line, ranging from half an inch to two inches in width, corresponding to the direction of the linea alba. The bellying recti muscles forming a ridge on either side, as the patient raised herself by their action, thus demonstrated the extent of this abnormal chink. In all the cases examined I found evidence of previous pregnancy or miscarriage, the abdominal parietes being always thin and muscular, and the whole frame rather wiry than obese. Evidence of displacement occurred in only five out of the fifteen cases, and in these the splitting of tissue between the recti muscles, which constituted the remarkable chink described, could not be traced to hold any relation to the uterine displacement. Indeed, in only one of the fifteen cases had the patient noticed that there was any peculiarity in her abdomen. Whether such a condition is congenital or always acquired remains yet to be ascertained.

In all these cases of mechanical influence from without, the sustentative structures which surround the uterus may suffice to restore its healthy position, provided that there do not exist other and more important conditions which either overcome or tend to annul their natural elastic action. But it usually happens that the causes which immediately induce or lead up to such an unfavourable state exercise a twofold operation; increasing the weight of the uterus itself, either of the whole organ or some part of it, and at the same time diminishing the healthy condition of the connective structures around. The deviations from the natural order of place which are thus produced find their most frequent and most marked illustrations in cases of prolapsus.

PROLAPSUS, or procidentia, includes those disorders of place, where the whole uterus is bodily depressed from its natural position. It comprises a wide variety of conditions;—which may still be considered together, in so far as they all, more or less, represent an alteration of those provisions arranged for the maintenance of its order of place. In extent the prolapsus may vary from a slight external pouting of the recto or vesico-vaginal mucous membranes up to so extreme a protrusion, that the uterus touches the ground when the woman is placed on her knees. But the extent of extra-vulval protrusion is of less importance than the recognition of the elements which compose it, and the discrimination of the manner of its production.

In prolapsus there may occur every conceivable variation in the adjustment of the two important agencies (the dynamic and vascular) described when considering the order of place; either may be disarranged, or both may be in fault.

In prolapsed vagina, the external protrusion may in size and shape resemble two oranges placed one over the other; the os uteri just coming into view between them. In a well-defined case of this kind, the womb may be of the natural size and length, and its structure healthy. It has simply followed the vagina in its descent, constituting a prolapsus dependent on a yielding of the sustentative structure; the uterus itself having nothing to do with the process. This may be denominated *passive* prolapsus uteri.

In contrast with such cases are those which represent the most frequent form of true prolapsus uteri; itself the most frequent kind of displacement. Here the beginning of the evil is an increase in size and weight of the organ. Its length may be more than double that found in health, and its walls present a corresponding increase in volume, though the structure be of diminished consistence, lax and spongy, and readily bleeding if the sound be too roughly introduced within the elongated cavity. Such a physical condition of the organ is not unfrequently met with in multiparæ, especially at the commencement of the change of life, or where the involution after parturition has not been duly accomplished. But in these latter cases, as during the advancement of pregnancy, increase in weight and size of the womb does not, of necessity, induce displacement.

We may consider as cases of *active* prolapsus those where the organ is large, and its increased weight induces displacement. But the same relaxed and enfeebled habitude which most frequently conduces to this condition degrades also the sustaining power of the connective structures. That which is true of a part is true of the whole body. There is a general enfeeblement and sluggish fulfilment of all the functions of life; Even the effort to withstand any of the ordinary influences of gravitation is more than can be borne, the veins of the legs swelling and the ankles becoming puffed as the day advances.

This active prolapsus uteri most frequently occurs in multiparæ, and generally dates its commencement from miscarriage, or confinement, followed by some defective involution of the uterus. That in these cases the liver should be disordered, the portal venous system engorged, and the uterus in some sort act as an indirect diverticulum of the venous blood may be understood from the described relations between the portal and uterine venous system. The weight which the uterus thus acquires is not met by any increase of sustaining power; so it gradually forces before it the yielding vagina, and displaces the adjacent organs by the strain of its continuous drag—the vagina being inverted from above. The history of such a case may extend over months or years; the external protrusion being finally determined by some vehement strain, such as the effort to lift a heavy weight; or by the indirect influence of some hepatic disorder and portal obstruction, to which the patient refers all her suffering. It has been said that "prolapsus, with the exception of certain rare cases of violence, or complicated with morbid growths, can only take place in the uterus which has undergone parturition."[1] There have, however, come under my notice two well-marked cases in which there was every indication of virginity; in addition to the os uteri being round and smooth. In each case the cervix protruded between the labia; and in one of them, æt. 27, there was a smooth continuous duplicature of

---

[1] Dr. Rigby's Diseases of Women, p. 130.

the hymeneal membrane distinctly raised from the surface of the canal, quite different from the caruncular appearance produced by forcible rupture. The history of the case favoured the opinion that the woman was a virgin.

As prolapsus, dependent on uterine engorgement, or increase of weight, takes advantage of a co-existent deficiency in the true sustaining structures, and is only produced when these are enfeebled or strained beyond endurance, so also the rectum and bladder only force out the corresponding parts of the vagina when the natural supporting power is abrogated.

On such a view of the Pathology of Prolapsus, it is evident that the introduction of wooden rings and other contrivances for dilating the vagina, and thus supporting the uterus, can have but a very limited efficiency, and may even do harm rather than good. It was, until very recently, the custom to introduce large boxwood pessaries, which were often worn for months together. Sometimes they effected a cure, the pressure on the vaginal plexus relieving the strain on the uterine veins. But if, coincident with this, no relief was afforded to the portal congestion, then ascites was not unfrequently produced, the veins of the portal system being relieved by peritoneal exudation, as in ordinary cases of obstructive liver disease. And sometimes the local influence exercised by these pessaries led to good or harm in other ways. Long continued local pressure on the walls of the vagina produced ulceration; and so large were the instruments used, that occasionally the solid wood had to be broken into fragments to allow of its extraction before the ulceration could be treated. After this had been effected, cicatrisation was followed by so much contraction of the calibre of the vagina, that protrusion no longer occurred. And it was this natural process of contraction during cicatrisation which first suggested the removal of a part of the vaginal mucous membrane as a curative operation for prolapsus. In other cases the result was far more serious, since the continual intra-vaginal pressure set up inflammation, and led to pelvic cellulitis and to death.

The objections to the wooden rings employed as pessaries for the last five hundred years, apply, in a modified degree, to the numerous modern instruments devised for restoring and retaining in place the prolapsed uterus. They are too often used, much as a truss is applied in cases of hernia, to insure temporary relief rather than to assist in the establishment of a radical cure. The value of a pessary is to maintain the displaced organs in position, so that an opportunity may be afforded for unimpeded action of those agencies which maintain the Order of Place in Health. The use of an instrument is only ancillary to that treatment which has for its object the removal of the original cause of the disorder of place.

The treatment of the *passive form* of prolapsus uteri, where the organ follows a protrusion of the vagina, requires that attention be exclusively given to the latter condition. The disorder itself occurs under two forms. In one, laceration of the perineum having occurred during labour, there gradually ensues a protrusion of the posterior and anterior walls, carrying with them pouches of the adjacent hollow organs, and forming respectively vaginal rectocele and cystocele. The former protrusion is usually the most marked, and may even occur without the rectum being implicated, since the attachments to the gut are far more lax than those which exist between the vagina and bladder. But where the rectum is pouched into the vagina, the finger readily passes forwards into the hollow on an anal examination being made. In such cases, that plastic procedure, known as the " perineal operation," affords a simple and efficient means of permanent cure, since it directly remedies the cause of the protrusion. In the second form of passive prolapsus the perineum may be tolerably firm yet the protrusion be very large (*see* p. 48). Here also it may be necessary, in extreme cases, to resort to operative procedure, adopting the suggestion of Dr. Marshall Hall, to dissect off a part of the vaginal mucous membrane, and bring the edges together; but the instances are very rare where such extreme measures are required.

In the majority of cases, the treatment is suggested by attention to the causes of the protrusion, and the method may be best illustrated by a case.

E. J., æt. 22, a healthy-looking woman, unmarried, virginity doubtful, never pregnant, menstruation always regular, bowels habitually costive. Has a prolapsus vaginæ, the rectal and vesical walls so protruding as to resemble two tennis balls in size; with the cervix uteri just showing between. The prolapsus has gradually increased for two years. As the protrusion always went up at night, she did not seek advice until compelled by the increasing irritability of the bladder. By costiveness, she means that the exigencies of her work (chiefly standing, or carrying heavy weights upstairs) prevented her relieving either bowels or bladder when she felt occasion; and this retention became a habit. Never thought of attributing her ailment to this cause. She has felt the want of support, and so has worn a steel busk in her stays. She has for years suffered from leucorrhœa, but not to such an extent as to make her go to a doctor.

In this case, the woman's life was of such kind, that if the healthiest person were exposed to a similar condition, the same result might be predicated. The vaginal membrane soddened in leucorrhœal discharge, the bladder and rectum only relieved when loaded beyond endurance, the abdominal organs pressed down by the diaphragm working vicariously to the constricted ribs—all conduced to the same end. The treatment consisted in entire removal of the costal pressure, ordering that the rectum should be emptied each day by a cold enema, and the bladder relieved every four hours. A hip-bath of cold salt water to be used for a quarter of an hour each morning, and local astringents injected. In a fortnight the urgent symptoms had disappeared, but there still remained a considerable protruding of the recto-vaginal tissue, that of the vesical part being less prominent. As in these cases it is the bladder symptoms which usually produce the chief distress, the relief was more apparent than real. The use of alum and tannin suppositories and of an air-ball pessary afforded but temporary benefit; I therefore painted the surface with perchloride of iron, dissolved in equal parts of glycerine. Three days after, there was just a superficial erosion of the mucous membrane, but with a very slight amount of pain. As the sore contracted, the protrusion ceased. Two months afterwards she called on me with no perceptible evidence of protrusion, even when she strained vehemently.

This was an extreme case; but local applications have been so beneficial in many other instances, that their employment is here mentioned, as preferential to the use of the knife, or, at all events, worthy of trial before resorting to operation. In ordinary cases the use of an air-ball pessary for re-adjustment, followed by astringent suppositories, usually suffices to cure, provided that there be adopted for the relief of any unnatural extra-uterine strain, such means as were employed in this case.

Prolapsus of the uterus, originally dependent on a " bearing down" of the organ itself,—above referred to as *active* prolapsus—involves other causes, and requires considerable modifications in the treatment. Increase of volume and weight of the uterus is originally due to some disturbance in the natural order of circulation. The varying conditions of the uterine blood-supply have been already mentioned in describing the order of place, and have to be presently considered in reference to the order of function. But it may be here noted that congestion of the uterus, involving an inordinate amount of present blood in its tissue, differs widely from that state of active hyperæmia which marks a condition of congestion of the stomach, the lungs, or the kidneys. In these latter, when the capillaries are engorged, the life and action of the part is endangered. In the uterus, the large and internexed veins with the plexus that lie without its walls, may become loaded with blood moving but very sluggishly; yet the organ itself shall present no other indications of protest than is afforded by the mechanical influence of its increased weight.

Such a condition, preceding the occurrence of active uterine prolapsus, owes its recognition to the employment of the uterine sound as a means of diagnosis. We are thus enabled to measure the length of the uterus and the thickness of its walls, to judge as to the presence of irregular developments, abnormal growths, or intrinsic deviations of place. The enlargement of the organ in active prolapsus also induces other evils; for the emergent vessels of the uterine plexus pass between the folds of the broad ligament. If these are dragged on, the surfaces are proportionably coarcted, and the vessels which pass between the layers of serous membrane have their area of conduction diminished. Moreover, the increased weight unduly tries the strength of that distributed sustentative arrangement already described.

In the majority of cases of active uterine prolapsus, and especially where they are of long duration, pessaries afford but temporary benefit, the displacement recurring on their withdrawal, if the treatment does not extend beyond merely mechanical restoration of place. So far as its immediate effect is concerned, the pessary is a very valuable assistance towards treatment. But the numerous contrivances adapted to support the prolapsed uterus are really only evidences of ingenuity—modifications of less perfect devices adapted with the same object, and all failing to fulfil anything beyond the range of their immediate action. In an extreme case of prolapsus uteri, where the organ protrudes beyond the vulva to the size of a child's head, the various elastic and ball pessaries are of very little avail; and in many cases of merely internal uterine procidentia, where these are commonly ordered, there is in reality little necessity for any local appliance whatever.

It is evident that in uterine protrusion, dependent on active mechanical influence exercised by the enlarged and weighty womb, the first indication should be to insure its retention so far within the pelvis that a diminution of its bulk may be effected by restoration of the natural action of its vascular arrangement. To procure this result, the best form of pessary is that with two expanding wings, and which is known as "the butterfly," or Zwancke's pessary. It completes the bony arch by filling up the intra-pubic space, allowing the bladder and rectum to act, whilst it sustains the uterus within the pelvis; and thus it bears the weight of the organ, relieves the drag on the broad ligaments, and insures a period of rest, and for recovery of tone, to each of those threads of connective tissue which are so dragged on in an extreme case of true prolapsus uteri. The perfect form of this instrument is here represented :—

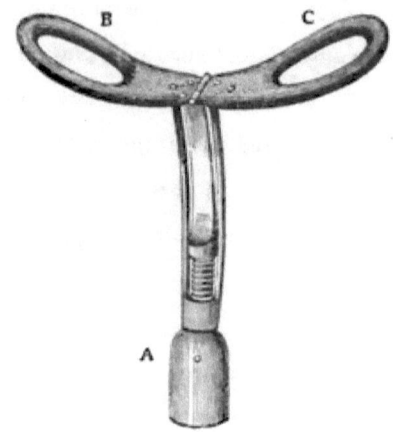

Dr. Simson, of St. Andrews, devised the first hinged pessary early in the last century.[1] Some fifty years later Schwenche[2] adopted the principle, and invented an instrument long known as his pessary. But he used a supported vaginal stalk, with the alæ expanding at its summit. This method has been recently re-introduced, having an india-rubber ball or cup in place of the dilating wings.

The preliminary restoration of place being effected, whatever the instrument used to maintain the advantage, there remain to be considered the indications of treatment which will insure a natural preservation of this order of place, and enable the patient to dispense with artificial aid.

Referring to my own notes of cases, I find in the vaginal

A, a handle which serves to expand the instrument after introduction; B, C represent the expanded alæ impeding by their action the descent of the uterus. The whole instrument should be made of vulcanite india-rubber.

[1] Edin. Med. Essays and Observations, vol. iii. p. 288.
[2] Comment. de Rebus in Scient. Nat. et Med. Leipsicæ, 1763.

and uterine prolapsus, as already distinguished, a marked difference as regards the hepatic condition and state of the portal circulation. In the former, the cause is usually localized to the vaginal tissues and its surroundings; in the latter, the uterine engorgement, ascertained by the touch and use of the sound, usually coincides with an amount of portal derangement which helps to explain the physical condition of the uterus on the data already given. The successful treatment in cases of acute prolapsus necessarily requires a diminution of the weight of the uterus. Wherever this weight depends upon a partial stasis of blood within the tissue, and where this has for its cause a retardation or obstruction of the portal circulation, with the coincident conditions already described, the course to be pursued for remedying the evil is evident. I omit from present consideration those cases of added growths, or intra-abdominal pressure, which involve special structural change, and all obvious mechanical influences—tight stays, heavy petticoats, straining efforts, and whatever causes irregular vesical or rectal pressure.

I sought some means of assisting or stimulating the action of the portal system, where its obstruction forms the original source of the trouble. The medicinal agent I selected and have largely employed is the hydrochlorate of ammonia. It is administered with the intention of immediate absorption into the portal venules which ramify beneath the surface of the digestive tract. It was first suggested by the results of certain well-known experiments on blood-stasis of the effects produced by injections and administration of different salts, and by a consideration of the recorded influence and mode of action of the drug, which has been for many years commonly employed in Germany as a deobstruent.

The use of hydrochlorate of ammonia for the purpose indicated implies a recognition of its value generally as an important agent for the relief of hepatic portal congestion. This I believe to be very great, but only one result of such congestion has to be here considered. Mercury, podophylline, taraxacum, aloes, &c., may be resorted to with the same intent in cases suitable for their employment. But in the following instances, selected because subsequent opportunities enabled me to verify the permanence of the result, the treatment was exclusively based on the administration of the hydrochlorate of ammonia, aided by those regulations as to hygienic treatment which have been described, and which are of such importance that the best devised medical treatment will fail unless they be observed.

HISTORY.	TREATMENT.
1. S. W., æt. 60, thin and worn. Prolapsus commenced 5 years ago; carried heavy weights, felt her strength diminish, so wore a steel busk and laced herself up "for the sake of the support." Uterus gradually protruded more and more, and now extrudes to the size of a turkey's egg—cervix large, granular erosion round the os as large as a florin.	Sore touched with solution of iodide of silver. Prolapse reduced and supported by a ball of oiled wool. A Zwancke's pessary introduced below this. Ammon. hydrochl. c. Tinct. ferri sesquichl. ordered three times a day. In a week the sore was healed. The pessary was worn for a fortnight, the medicine continued six weeks. No prolapse or suffering during this time. Four months afterwards had experienced no return of symptoms; and the uterus was diminished in size, natural in position, and the cervix healthy.

HISTORY.

2. M. T., æt. 56, florid, stout woman, had eight children, always suffered from bearing down for upwards of a month after confinements. Change of life five years ago, gradually increasing prolapsus ever since. Uterus protrudes as large as an orange. Has used instruments, which were either forced out or caused such pain that they had to be removed. Habit always constipated; subject to "bilious attacks" all her life. Membrane of cervix thickened, no erosion, sound passed to three and a quarter inches.

3. E. A., æt. 38, three miscarriages, two children born alive. Since last confinement has been "constantly ailing" and weak; menstruates regularly, but with great forcing pain, severe pruritus, and constant irritability of bladder. The os uteri, large and soft, presents between the labia, the vesical and rectal walls of vagina so protruding as to conceal the organ. The uterus advances outwards nearly an inch on a straining effort being made. Much acid dyspepsia.

4. E. G., æt. 48, 11 children, 3 miscarriages, menses ceased nine years ago, was ailing for five years previously. Reverse of circumstances, anxiety, and much nursing (having to frequently lift a sick husband) preceded the prolapsus, which first appeared externally three years ago, and has gradually become worse, protruding as large as a tennis ball, but receding altogether during the night—has had hæmorrhoids for two years. Cervix and uterus large.

TREATMENT.

Uterus returned; Zwancke's pessary introduced; great care in diet enjoined. Powder of sulphate of manganese and sulphate of magnesia every morning. Cold douche at night after removal of pessary, and hip-bath in morning. Hydrochlorate of ammonia, hydrochloric acid, and taraxacum three times a day. The prolapse did not recur; the pessary was left off after a month. Two years afterwards there had been no recurrence of displacement.

A well-filled air pessary introduced. An injection of lead and belladonna every morning. Rhubarb and soda until the digestion improved; subsequently ammon. hydrochl. with calumba, and Plummer's pill on alternate nights. The air-ball pessary was twice forced out during the first week, but afterwards retained. She ceased attendance in three weeks, as the symptoms had all disappeared. After three months she became again pregnant, with some return of the pruritus, but no prolapsus.

Uterus returned, Zwancke's pessary applied. Treatment as in Case 2. Tannin and belladonna ointment for piles. Three weeks afterwards reported that there had been no protrusion, but a sense of dragging when the instrument was left off. A fortnight after this was allowed to gradually leave off the pessary. Reported herself cured, and returned to the country in following week.

HISTORY.	TREATMENT.
5. A. M., æt. 52, suffered from bearing down since change of life four years ago, when she had several severe attacks of menorrhagia; cannot walk now from the constant pressure in body. Thin and sallow, subject to hepatic congestion all her life, "especially before poorly times;" always menstruated very freely; bowels constipated. Uterus just seen at vulva covered by a vesical protrusion; none of posterior vaginal wall.	Zwancke's pessary, manganese and magnesia in the morning; ammon. hydrochl. and tinct. ferri sesquichl., with quassia and chloric ether. Twelve days afterwards walked a mile without suffering; left off treatment, had a relapse with increase of all her original symptoms. After resuming treatment, she was enabled to get about in a fortnight, but was two months before the medicine could be discontinued.
6. T. D., æt. 53, a stout, florid woman; ten children; change of life six years ago; has suffered from a sense of bearing down ever since. The uterus first appeared externally three years ago, and now protrudes as large as an orange. She was a cook until middle life, subsequently kept a laundry, with constant standing and much hard work.	Treatment as above, with hip baths in morning. In a month (the uterus not having prolapsed) she left off the pessary, continuing the medicine. After two years she reported she had been "quite tight ever since," and without any sense of bearing down, though frequently turning a mangle for several hours a day.

In prolapsus uteri, comprising under this term all the varieties of delapsion already described, the cavity of the organ does not necessarily deviate from its natural direction. Though the cervix may present at the vulva, yet intra-uterine exploration by a bougie so prepared as to show, on withdrawal, the direction it has taken, will indicate that the gentle curve from os to fundus is still maintained; for the organ has just followed that course which in health is presented by the vaginal canal.

In the forms of uterine displacement next in frequency to prolapsus, the organ may retain its elevation within the pelvis, and the vaginal canal be natural in length and direction; for the deviation occurs above the superior pelvic fascia, and within the true pelvis. It may consist of an entire displacement of the uterus; its parts still maintaining their natural relation to each other, and the whole organ being more or less turned, like a pear on its stalk. To this condition the term " version of the uterus" should be exclusively restricted. Or the womb may be bent on itself, with a necessary alteration of the angle which the cervix forms with the fundus uteri: this constitutes flexion. In versions, the bending is at the top of the vagina; in flexions proper, it is in or above the uterine cervix.

Of these two conditions of disorder of place, that most frequently met with is uterine flexion. But this includes a wide range of displacement, ranging from a slight increase of the natural curve to a state in which the uterus is doubled down upon itself, and its cavity becomes bent like a hook. Curvature of the uterus to such an extent as to constitute a disorder of place, occurs most frequently in the direction forwards. Where the uterus is folded on itself at an acute angle, the fundus usually has its directions downwards and backwards, constituting retroflexion. The curvature forwards of the fundus uteri may exist to such an extent that the whole organ is bent like a crescent. Monsieur Valleix has especially directed attention to this condition; and its frequency, judging from my own experience, justifies special consideration of the conditions under which it arises.

ANTEFLEXION.—The purpose subserved by the close attachment of the superior part of the vagina, and inferior part of the body of the uterus to the posterior wall of the bladder, has been already mentioned. In childhood, and before the body of the uterus has undergone development, this attachment exercises a comparatively greater influence on the position of the uterus, producing that curvature forwards which represents the natural position of the undeveloped organ. Persistence of this condition represents a deficiency of uterine development in that which forms the adult contribution to its length. Such a deviation from the natural direction of the adult uterus may be distinguished as congenital anteflexion. It includes many, and probably the majority, of those numerous cases where ante-curvature of the uterus has been found after death without the occurrence of notable symptoms during life. Hence the assumption has been drawn, that deviations forwards of the uterus do not necessarily present those serious symptoms which practical observers have accredited to them. Such cases, on investigation, usually present a history of scanty menstrual flow, unaccompanied with suffering throughout virgin life; the whole of the correlative generative endowments having the same developmental deficiency of structure and function as the uterus itself. If the woman live and die a virgin, the post-mortem shows that her life has sexually been little in advance of that which obtains in childhood. But matrimony brings suffering. The function of the generative cycle is stimulated by the change of duties. The position of uterus is altered, its free cervix moving upwards and backwards, so that the condition approaches that of anteversion of the womb; the undeveloped body of the organ retaining its original connexions and tendency to curvature. If pregnancy ensue, the uterine changes then determined may make up for the retarded development. Sometimes the woman only suffers acutely throughout the early primiparous months. Or abortion may result from the double effort necessary to provide for uterine development and fœtal nourishment. In the latter case, that healthy determination which induces the reparative conditions known as uterine involution may set all right; so that the second pregnancy completes its course.

Some such history comprises, I believe, a large number of those cases where women, whose menstruation and sexual development is in arrear of their time of life, are said to be cured by marriage; an early miscarriage and much previous suffering preceding a second pregnancy, the subsequent uterine life being that of a healthy woman. Prolapsus uteri occurs most frequently among poor and hard-worked women. The deviation of place now under consideration, depending primarily on deficient sexual and uterine development, is chiefly met with among those who are nursed in the lap of luxury, and reared with an utter disregard of their future physical well-being.

There are thus presented two conditions under which the ante-curved uterus of childhood may come to assume its full development and due relation of place. 1st. By the natural changes determined at puberty. 2nd. By the process of uterine renewal which follows any reproductive effort. There are also two conditions under which the congenital condition of ante-curvature is persistent. 1st. In the virgin, where a whole life may pass without trouble or suffering. 2nd. In the married woman, where no proportional uterine development ensues, and where matrimonial life is a misery. The catamenia do not increase, nor do the sexual conditions alter, but there gradually ensue symptoms which denote displacement forwards of the womb, with constant dragging pain, irritability of the bladder, extreme abdominal tenderness, and an increasing inability to walk, to undergo exertion, or even to maintain, for long together, a standing position.

Such cases present a foregone history, to which the local examination affords a clue. The os uteri is high up in the pelvis; the cervix is usually less developed than in health, and very tender to the touch; and the body of the organ may be simply curved forwards, or even be felt lying in front of, or sharply bent on, the cervix. Anteflexion of the uterus may ensue from other causes; the development of interstitial deposits in its anterior walls, the presence of tumours, the occurrence of such entire want of textural tone that the organ weighs down on the bladder as it fills, and follows its collapse on micturition. But in all these cases the cervix is lower than usual in the canal, whereas in the class of cases above described it is always more distant than in health, and may have been so far urged upwards, that the os uteri is reached with difficulty by the finger of an expert. Moreover, in congenital anteflexion the distance from os to fundus, as measured by the sound, is usually below the average; in cases of anteflexion dependent on other causes, it usually exceeds the normal length.

With the patient lying on her side, well coiled up, and having the bladder emptied, the recognition of anteflexion of the womb is comparatively easy, and the position of the cervix assists the diagnosis as to its cause. But the introduction of the sound affords the only absolutely reliable information, since tumours within or in front of the anterior uterine wall, and felt through the roof of the vagina, may simulate displacement. Indeed, in all cases of flexion and of pelvic tumour, the direction of the uterine cavity must be ascertained before any decision can safely be given. A previous tactile examination affords to an expert information by which he regulates the curve of the sound. Thus, in severely ante-cornuate uteri it may be impossible to introduce an instrument having the usual curve, and passed in the usual direction; but if the sound be made to enter the cervix with its concavity backwards, it may then be gently turned, so that the point will readily pass forwards into the hooked hollow of the fundus, affording a guide both as to the direction, extent, and regularity of the intra-uterine cavity.

ANTEVERSION.—In describing the active form of prolapsus uteri, reference has been made to a class of patients with sluggish circulation and little physical energy, who are deficient in vitality, and in whom prolapsus represents only a local symptom of some general failure in vigour. It may be that after long wear and tear the woman has " broken up," as it is expressively phrased; or that a life of indolence, without the exercise necessary to stimulate reparation of tissue, has borne its fruits in an early loss of the reparative power. Among the poor of great cities this thorough state of dilapidation not unfrequently presents itself even at an early age; and it is eminently necessary to primarily recognise the general defect instead of directing attention to the treatment of the local affection.

In such cases the uterus is usually large and soft and heavy; but without heat or tenderness or tendency to lesion. Any or all of these may be readily produced by undue interference, and any such local treatment is certain to do harm. In persons thus vitally deficient, the heavy uterus may deviate in any direction, according to the action of influences from without. It is thus that anteversion most frequently occurs, the organ being displaced forwards in the whole length of its body, with the cervix turned backwards. There is little suffering beyond a constant sense of drag, which is relieved by the recumbent posture. The pendulous abdominal walls, often loaded with fat, no longer afford due support, and allow the bladder to distend, sometimes to an inordinate extent; its sudden emptying serving to increase the anteversion. It is when approaching the era of change, and when the anteversion has become considerable, that, as Dr. Chambers remarks, " many wives lose suddenly the inclination for, and the power to bear their matrimonial privileges." It is in such cases, the catamenia becoming deficient or ceasing, and the flabby uterus affording a feeling of increased weight, that the patient often comes to suspect herself pregnant, and may even carry on this conviction to the extent of preparing for her confinement. In these cases very great care should be used in the employment of the sound. Its use is, of course, entirely out of the question, should there be the least reason to suspect pregnancy. But where the uterus is large and soft, approaching that condition which Rokitansky designates as pulpiness, a very slight urging of the instrument might cause it to penetrate the softened uterine walls. This has been frequently done, so that the sound has passed almost to its handle. Luckily, the tendency to sthenic inflammation is not great in these cases ; but the easy passage of the instrument is no indication that it may with impunity be urged as far as it will penetrate. Such a condition of the womb may lead to other ills. If the structural debility be somewhat less than that described, the mechanical changes ensuing on impregnation may eventually induce displacement of the whole organ, so as to set up expulsive action, thus producing recurring abortions. Or the debilitated organ may become partially introverted, the fundus settling down within the cup formed by the non-resistant walls of the cavity, a condition especially noted by Dr. Rigby as producing what he called the squatting uterus.

If the large and ill-renovated uterus, either by constant recumbence or natural position, assumes a position in which its fundus is turned backwards, then the urging of a loaded rectum with the expulsive effort made to obtain relief, may at any time force down the fundus into the cavity of the sacrum, sometimes causing true retroversion, but most generally producing that displacement which constitutes retroflexion of the womb, when its fundus can be distinctly felt in the space of Douglas, and the sharp bend at or about the depth of the internal os may be readily distinguished.

Before considering cases of retroflexion originating in this way, it is necessary to refer to the important influence of displacements forwards in determining repeated abortions. Where such untoward events occur again and again in the same woman, it is eminently unsatisfactory to fall back on the old idea that the uterus, when distended to the size which it attains about the twelfth week of pregnancy, contracts a vicious habit of expelling its contents, that there is somehow developed a liability to the occurrence of such mishaps; and that the patient's best chance of tiding over the evil time is to keep very quiet, physically and mentally; the result of which is, that the bodily inaction impairs her physical strength, and the mental rest induces a morbid contemplation of the threatening danger.

In cases of the kind here alluded to, it is very important to ascertain by digital examination the position of the uterus, at the earliest opportunity; and, if deviation be discovered, to remedy the disorder of place, carefully watching the movements of the womb until it has risen out of the pelvis. If the displacement of the increasing uterus be backwards, there ensue a series of symptoms which give ample warning and indicate the necessity for reposition ; whether the fundus has been, as it were, caught by the sacral promontory, or an original deviation has increased as the body of the uterus becomes more weighty. This cause of uterine expulsive action has been carefully described. Its symptoms are urgent, and afford previous warning of the danger which threatens. But where the uterus, as its weight and bulk increase, topples forwards and produces anteversion, there need occur no special symptoms prior to those which indicate that expulsive action has commenced, and the mischief is done. Now the first result of that effort is to insure that the womb tends to reassume its normal direction. So that when the practitioner is summoned, the organ is found in its place, and the case presents all the characters of an ordinary *fausse-couche*. I have notes of three cases in which such a condition of anteversion had been probably the cause of many previous miscarriages. In two of them there was distinct anteversion of the uterus. One had previously miscarried three, and the other four, successive times. One I saw at the eighth, and the other at the tenth week of pregnancy. In both there were symptoms of irritability of the bladder, which led me to question more closely. They had both been thus troubled when previously pregnant (one had borne living children), and they looked on these symptoms as natural to the parturient state. In the third case, the patient summoned me because of certain sensations which she had, by experience, learnt to consider as harbingers of "another trouble." The uterus, in this instance, was considerably anteverted, and expulsive action commencing; here miscarriage occurred. In the two cases first mentioned, the patients carried their young to the full time.

The expedients adopted comprised a gentle replacement of the womb, the vaginal finger urging the cervix, the other hand being placed on the abdomen to gently assist the movement of the uterus; turning it, as it were, on its axis. Every source of pressure from above was removed, and the lower abdominal zone supported by a firm belt, having a pad of curled horsehair on the anterior part.[1] Exercise was enjoined, exertion forbidden; the bladder was emptied at regular hours—unless occasion required its being sooner done—and straining of every kind was prohibited. The practical point which has induced this digression, is the importance of examining the position of the uterus early in pregnancy, wherever miscarriage has previously occurred; so as to recognise and remedy that disorder of place which frequently foregoes the commencement of expulsive effort.

DISPLACEMENTS BACKWARD are of very rare occurrence in the virgin uterus, except there be some neoplastic deposit, which, by mere weight, exercises a mechanical in-

---

[1] Dr. Hull's "Abdominal Support" is admirably adapted for cases of this nature.

fluence or evidence of some vehement jerks. The facility afforded by the extent of the vaginal pouch behind the cervix uteri, is here counterbalanced by the occasional presence of tumours, which present to the touch very much the character of retroflexion; the cervix occupying its ordinary place and direction, and a rounded tumour felt as lying between its upper part and the rectum. Thus, a dislocated ovary, or fibrous growths descending into the space of Douglas, abdominal tumours, hæmatoceles, or abscesses, may mislead if the touch is alone relied on.

True retroversion, with the uterus lying in a straight line across the pelvis, having its os directly forwards, is of rare occurrence. It may happen from a violent jerk, and cases have been recorded where even such an entire displacement of the pregnant uterus has yet not induced the usual expulsive action. It is far less frequently found than retroflexion, although a modified form of this altered direction of the whole organ probably precedes, in the majority of cases, those changes which finally establish true retroflexion of the organ. This especially happens under the conditions of impaired general health, already frequently referred to, where the uterus is large, heavy, and soft, and the sound indicates that it exceeds the natural length; this measurement of excess being in all probability sometimes due to the pressure of the instrument, so that the increased length is obtained by a diminution of the breadth. Such a state of atony of uterine muscular fibre occurs in all women under certain conditions, and to a modified extent at all periods of renewal of its tissue, when new structure replaces that which has fulfilled its purpose. After each pregnancy there is such an entire renovation, the uterus being, during its time of involution, in an atonic state. With each catamenial period there occurs, in a lesser degree, a similar reparation of tissue.

That enfeebled and atonic condition of the uterine structure, which commonly precedes retroflexion of the organ, generally originates in some arrest or deficiency of nutritive changes. Sometimes the state of the general health affords the clue; more frequently there is a distinct history, which traces back the commencement of the ailment to a period when the structure of the organ was yet in a transition state of reparation. Thus there may be an account of hard work, or sudden jerk soon after a lingering labour, or of successive miscarriages ensuing rapidly, or of some vehement strain made before the catamenia had ceased; or there is a history of violent effort by one who presents those general evidences of malnutrition already described.

The most important consideration in all cases of retroflexion, is in reference to the general state of health. The diagnosis of the displacement may be simple, but the method of its treatment, and the assurance of permanent reposition, depends upon a prior recognition of the original conditions which allowed the deviation of place; for a perfectly healthy uterus is a firm structure and able to hold its own, nor does it double back on itself under any such ordinary effort as suffices to produce retroflexion where the organ has lost its structural tonicity.

A displacement of the uterus is just as much an absolute fact as the occurrence of a hernial protrusion. The symptoms are well marked when properly investigated, and the relief afforded by reposition certifies the correctness of the diagnosis. It is one of the strong assertions of the extreme French school, that all the sufferings which attend and indicate uterine displacement, are to be explained by congestion or inflammation of the womb.[1] Those who maintain this doctrine have at least the merit of being very consistent in their views of uterine pathology, and very bold in their enunciation of them. My own experience, public and private, derived from close observation of a very large number of cases, compels me to dissent altogether from this view. It appears to me that the treatment of these cases for inflammation, neglecting reposition of the uterus, is about as erroneous as it would be to treat a strangulated hernia by leeching the sac, without attempting to replace the bowel. The considerations which govern the treatment when disorder of place has been ascertained to exist, comprise—

---

[1] These are the words of one of the latest writers—"The displacement theory is founded on a most fallacious assumption. I maintain with Lisfranc, P. Dubois, Depaul, Gosselin, Bennet, Remak, and Goupil, that with the exception of prolapsus uteri, uterine displacements have no proper symptoms, and that the pain and other symptoms that accompany them are to be explained by congestion or inflammation of the womb, of its mucous lining, or of its serous envelope."—Dr. Tilt on Uterine Therapeutics, 1864.

1st. The reposition of the organ.

2nd. The remedying of the conditions which originally led to, or tend to reproduce, deviation of position.

Whichever be the kind of uterine displacement, however extreme its extent, and whatever the proposed plan of treatment, the first indication is to produce restoration of the natural position, if this be possible; for there occur certain exceptional cases where it would be eminently injudicious to attempt any interference, on account of adhesions having been formed, binding down the displaced organ in its unnatural position.

Reposition of the retroflexed uterus, if the organ be bent to an extreme degree, can rarely be accomplished without the adept use of the sound. Where the displacement is less in degree, and recent, especially if the patient be thin, restoration may often be effected by steady digital pressure upwards and forwards of the displaced fundus; but this can only be thoroughly effected when the patient is two-thirds turned towards the prone position. The attempt at digital replacement should in every case be made. If not successful, the examination supplies accurate information as to the position, extent, and resistance of the displacement, as to the requisite curving of the sound, and the direction of its introduction.

The employment of this valuable instrument has been most unreasonably decried. It requires care and judgment in its use, for mischief may easily be done by handling it roughly, or attempting to overcome resistance by force. Properly employed, there is no danger in its introduction, whilst the information it is capable of affording is very valuable. Indeed, I believe that, in any hundred cases of uterine disorder or disease taken indiscriminately, one might far more safely dispense with the speculum than with the uterine sound. The educated touch can approximatively tell the condition of the cervix uteri; but such an extension of the finger as the sound supplies is essential for correct assurance as to the length, direction, and outline of the uterine cavity.

In a case of severe retroflexion, ascertained by tactile examination, the sound requires to be well curved, and to be introduced with its concavity towards the sacrum. The patient should be laid on her side, with the thighs bent towards the abdomen, whilst the operator guides the point of the sound into the cervix. From the time that this enters the os uteri attention should be directed chiefly to the position of its handle; the direction of its point can only be judged of, and influenced by, the movement of this handle.

As the finger gently urges up the displaced fundus, the curved sound gradually passes to the extremity of the cavity; and then the handle of the instrument, hitherto pointed backwards, moves easily, until it obtains a position more or less in a line with the body. At this stage, the cavity of the uterus, however distorted it may be, has the sound penetrating to its fundal depth; then the finger, hitherto lying behind the cervix, may be shifted to ascertain by the gauge at the back of the sound the length to which it has passed.

Such an introduction of the instrument to the full extent of the cavity of the displaced uterus is an essential preliminary to replacement. The stage next to that of thorough introduction is reposition of the womb; moving the fundus uteri upwards, forwards, and then somewhat downwards. This demands great care, for any undue strain may do considerable mischief. First, the handle of the sound must be shifted backwards (the intravaginal finger being pressed on the anterior part of the cervix, so that the instrument shall not recede); then the handle must be so moved that it gradually describes a half-circle, of which the axis is in the cervix (varying according to the extent of the curve), and the radius consists of the distance from this point to the extremity of the handle. This movement gradually lifts the fundus of the uterus on the extremity of the sound, so that it is not dragged towards the side, or subjected to a double curvature. The sweep of the stem of the instrument is so great, that it barely passes the back of the thigh when this is thoroughly bent on the abdomen. As the handle of the sound comes down it takes a direction forwards, lying eventually between the thighs. In this position (considering the original curve required for its introduction), the indication given by the sound is that the uterus is now replaced in its normal position.

I have thus described, at some length, the method of replacing a retroflexed uterus, not having met with any such detailed directions elsewhere. If, when the sound has penetrated to the depth of the retorted cavity, an effort were made to twist the instrument, making the handle an axis and whirling the uterus round, then it is perfectly explicable how the serious results recorded as evidence against the use of the sound have arisen. Any one holding a bent sound in his hand, and rotating it, will at once perceive what a powerful leverage is thus exercised; and how the uterus is dragged into a new condition of lateral deviation whilst undergoing the half-turn that is to bring its concavity forwards; with great probability of injuring the delicate tissues pressed on. *The only safe rule for reduction of all disorders of uterine place is, that the organ shall be gently caused to retraverse the course originally passed through on its way from the natural to the unnatural position.*

With replacement of the displaced uterus all symptoms sometimes cease. The two following cases illustrate such result :—

Mrs. A., æt. 43, stout, florid, married, with one child; menstruation natural until three months ago; then she fell downstairs and was much bruised. When able to get about, she experienced an unusual sense of weight in the body, with much dragging pain on either side. She persevered in her efforts to take exercise, but with constantly-increasing suffering. The pain extended down her legs, until she was compelled to walk in a bent position; a persistent white discharge came on, action of the bowels caused her intense suffering, her bladder became irritable, and at the menstrual periods she had a profuse and exhaustive flow, but without any relief to the pain. She had been ordered injections for the leucorrhœa, which arrested the discharge, but so increased the forcing pain that she had to omit their use. On examination I found the uterus low down, large, and firmly retroflexed, with the rounded fundus in the space of Douglas, and very tender. The organ was cautiously replaced, with only slight suffering, and the cervix brought well backwards. All weight of the dress and pressure from above was forbidden, a firm binder placed on the body, some days of absolute rest enjoined, and a cold sitz-bath daily. The lady lived some distance from town, and I did not see her again for a fortnight. All her sufferings ceased after the replacement. She had carefully avoided physical efforts until her journey to visit me; the uterus was in place, the body larger than natural, and the sound passing to the distance of nearly three inches without pain. Hydrochlorate of ammonia with hydrochloric acid and a bitter infusion was ordered three times a day, and observance of the golden rule, "avoid jerk." The following menstrual period was somewhat prolonged, but without pain, and the flow at no time excessive. Three months afterwards she called to announce her entire recovery.

Mrs. P., æt. 25, married six years, miscarried soon after marriage, with much subsequent suffering. For this she was treated during two years on the assumption that she had "uterine inflammation," was leeched frequently, had caustic applied, and "had so many things to attend to—douches, injections, physic, and liniments—that she used to become bewildered." I saw her first in 1862, when the cervix uteri was hard, nodulated, and tender, and the general health debilitated by her long suffering. She rapidly improved under the local application of iodine and internal administration of iron, and returned to the country. In 1864 she became pregnant, and had an easy labour. Fifteen months after she called to ask my advice as to some internal piles which had troubled her ever since her confinement, without any benefit being derived from treatment. She suffered from occasional bleeding per rectum, especially when the evacuations were hard. She had given up both walking and riding, for they increased the forcing sensation which had been, more or less, constantly present since she got up after her confinement. Menstruation ensued on weaning her child, five months previous to her visit, and the periods had been attended with increasing suffering. On examination, the fundus uteri was found to be curved backwards, not absolutely flexed, and the os uteri, though low down in the vagina, did not present forwards as in true retroversion. After replacements, the sensation of pressure backwards, the pain on defecation, and the passage of blood entirely ceased. The following menstrual period was unaccompanied by suffering, and she could walk and ride without experiencing any discomfort. She has since become pregnant. Here also there was considerable congestion of the uterus, due to unnatural strain and an original deficiency in the process of involution. The medicines ordered were the same as in the previous case.

But mere reposition of the displaced uterus, whether the original direction of its flexion was forwards or backwards, does not usually afford such ready results. If the replacement be well done, there is relief for a brief time, but the trouble will recur if the chronically flexed uterus be merely restored to its natural place, and then left without some extra support; since the wall of the organ has become atrophied and thin at the line of flexion. In severe and chronic cases of uterine flexion it is important to maintain in place the rehabilitated uterus, for the reason already referred to when describing the treatment of prolapsus; here also the mechanical treatment is only ancillary to the more important general treatment—is, in fact, only a temporary expedient. An infinity of instruments have been devised for the purpose of maintaining the uterus in its place—some vaginal, some intra-uterine. The extra-uterine pessaries of H. de Chegoin, of Dr. Hodges, and of Dr. Priestley, act by fitting behind the cervix, and being there so adapted to the curve of the sacrum as to impede the descent of the previously replaced fundus. But in a large number of cases the tissues behind the cervix have become so tender from long-continued pressure that these instruments cannot be borne. The vaginal stem pessaries, dilating the vagina or pressing up the cervix uteri, have not been found successful in practice; for where the flexion is chronic, the malposition of the fundus returns in despite of them. The air-ball vaginal pessary, as suggested by Valleix, is occasionally useful, especially where the uterus is large, and its posterior walls thickened by interstitial neoplastic deposit, as in the following case :—

Mrs. D., æt. 40, a widow, five years ago was suddenly roused by a night alarm, and for some time stood with her bare feet on the cold stone stairs. She was menstruating at the time; the menses were suddenly checked, and she suffered from subsequent metritis, with the formation of several pelvic abscesses. On getting about, she experienced all the symptoms of retroflexion. During three years she suffered very greatly on the least movement, with severe dysmenorrhœa and exhaustive menorrhagia at the periods, which were regular. She first came under my care on account of the intense headaches which accompanied the attacks throughout. *En passant*, I may mention that these were entirely relieved by galvanism, using the Faradisation apparatus. The uterus was bulky, the cervix large and somewhat hard, the os wide and curvilinear, its posterior lip being thickened, and forming the convexity of the curve. The fundus could be felt, like a tennis-ball, in the space of Douglas, and the sound indicated that the mass was chiefly due to a thickening of the posterior wall, forced down beneath the lumbo-sacral promontory. There were other complications, which interfered with any immediate reposition of the uterus. When this had been effected, and the direction of the womb turned well forwards, an india-rubber ball was fully dilated high up in the vagina—thus pressing the cervix upwards and backwards, the weight of the womb assisting the purpose, which was to produce a virtual anteversion. The success was complete. By general treatment the uterus was gradually diminished in bulk, and the patient, who had lain on her couch for upwards of two years slowly but entirely recovered, leaving off the air-ball pessary at the end of two months.

It was the proved inefficiency of extra-uterine pessaries in a large number of the most severe cases which suggested the application of an intra-uterine support, acting on the uterus like the stilette of a wax bougie, fixing and sustaining the cavity in its normal position by a firm stalk, which should prevent any forcible flexion of the organ; the uterus—thus supported by the intra-uterine pessary—being gradually repaired in those parts thinned by long flexion, or strained by an abnormal curvature. The principle of the treatment was excellent, but in practice it signally failed, and for the following reason. The uterus is never absolutely at rest, as already explained. It is endowed with a special irritability, causing expulsive effort when any point of its cavity is subjected to pressure, and if the attempt at eviction be not successful, local irritation soon goes on to inflammation, and there follows a history of metritis, and of pelvic inflammation, with all that serious train of symptoms which induced the strong condemnation of intra-uterine pessaries when their employment was discussed by the French Academy of Medicine.

When a stem of ivory or metal was placed within the uterus, with the intention that it should act like the intra-uterine portion of a carefully introduced sound, the expulsive action of the organ was found to gradually force it out of the cavity; so that the old displacement was soon reproduced. To obviate this result, Sir G. Y. Simpson affixed his intra-uterine stem to a firm support placed externally. Thus the fundus of the uterus, at each inspiration or effort, as of coughing, sneezing, &c., was forced down upon an unyielding, un-elastic, intra-uterine stilette, and such mechanical irritation soon produced serious results. In this way there ensued those injurious consequences which appear to have followed the use of Sir G. Y. Simpson's intra-uterine pessary in other hands than his own. His success is probably attributable to such careful adjustment of the instrument that it should be sufficiently far introduced to prevent the occurrence of flexion, and yet not be long enough to touch the fundus uteri. Valleix recognised the importance of this, and he alone appears to have met with such success as to warrant his speaking favourably of the use of this form of intra-uterine pessary.

The chief essentials for an efficient intra-uterine pessary are 1 :—that it shall not interfere with the movements of the uterus itself; and 2 :—shall not impinge upon, and exercise a lever power by pressure against, any point of the cavity of the replaced uterus. Two instruments have been suggested to meet these requirements, their intra-uterine retention being assured by their having such size as to dilate the cervix : the one consists of a curved metal tube, much resembling a large tracheal tube, the other is composed of an elastic coil of wire, in a flexible gutta-percha case. The want of success attending their use is attributable to the neglect of two other equally essential requirements. 3 : There must be no dilatation of the cervix, since this induces expulsive uterine effort. 4 : The weight of the instrument must cause no drag on the sustentative structures.

It was with full recognition of these difficulties that I devised my own instrument. There had come under my notice a number of those cases of retroflexion, where ordinary means of support are absolutely useless, and where the very serious results recorded as following on the introduction of the intra-uterine pessaries hitherto employed, might well deter the cautious practitioner from exposing the patient to such great risk.

It was essential for an efficient intra-uterine pessary, that it should not interfere with the movements of the organ itself, since these must go on. I recognised that only mischief could result from allowing the possibility of pressure against any one point of the intra-uterine surface ; that any continued dilatation of the cervix would certainly induce expulsive action, and that the only way in which physical elasticity could be safely counteracted was by elastic resistance.

My instrument for assuring the continuance in place of a flexed uterus resembles in appearance a short sound, having a guard-plate (A) at such distance from the extremity as to represent nearly the normal uterine length. After very careful replacement of the uterus, as already described, the instrument is introduced just as an ordinary sound until the guard comes to touch against the cervix, when the smoothly-rounded end (B) lies free within the cavity of the

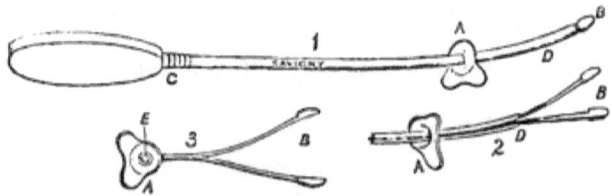

uterus, the intervening part being bent to the natural curve of the organ. The finger retains the guard-plate *in situ*, whilst the canula (C, D, figs. 1 and 2) is withdrawn. The spring-pessary expands, as shown in figs. 2 and 3, lying along each lateral wall of the intra-uterine cavity, as seen in fig. 4. The breadth of the spring prevents any antero-posterior flexion, and its elasticity antagonizes expulsive effort, whilst the movements of the uterus, as a whole, are in no way restricted. The withdrawal of the instrument is accomplished by introducing the canula until its point touches the hollow on the vaginal surface of the guard-plate, as seen in fig. 4. There is a slit on the back of the canula which receives the metal bar connecting the spring with the guard-plate. Thence it readily glides into the collar, and collapses the spring, as in fig. 1. There is no need to employ the speculum either for introduction or withdrawal.

It was my original intention that the intra-uterine spring

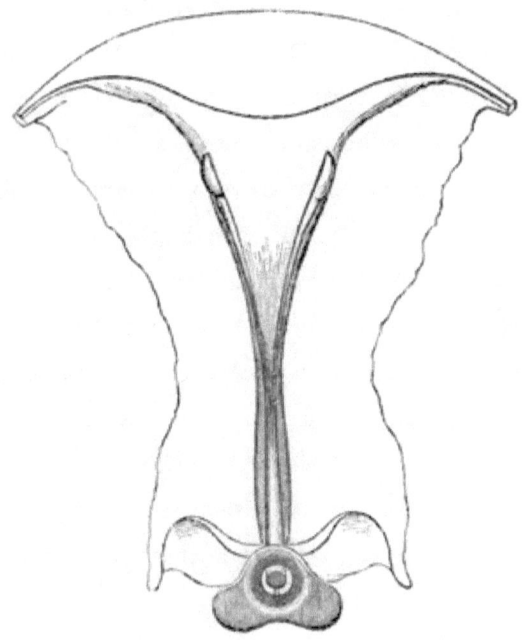

Fig. 4.

should be plated with gold, but I have found in practice that the steel merely becomes smoothly covered with a black sulphuret, and undergoes no further change, even when retained for a fortnight. The length of the spring employed should be judged from previous exploration by the sound. The canula allows the intra-uterine pessary to be of any length required; that usually employed measures two inches and a sixth.[1]

There is no novelty in the use of an intra-uterine spring. It was first employed by Dr. Martin Wear in 1855, whose instrument was again introduced into notice by Dr. Balandin of St. Petersburgh, in 1865. Several other adaptations have been suggested, but all of them failing to fulfil those requirements noted as essential to success in the use of an intra-uterine pessary to remedy flexions of the uterus.

LATERAL DISPLACEMENT OF THE UTERUS may depend on original want of bilateral symmetry in development of the organ, or be due to some neoplastic deposit occupying only one side of the uterus. It may be induced by pressure from without, as during the growth of an ovarian or other tumour; but it occurs most frequently, and must continue to occur, wherever pelvic cellulitis, confined to one side, has gone on to the production of abscess. If the patient recover after evacuation of the purulent matter, and from that great drain on the system produced by frequent re-accumulation, the method of healing is much the same as in other parts where abscess has formed among the meshes of areolar tissue. There follows contraction; the extent of which, after pelvic abscess of one side, determines how far the uterus is drawn from its central position. In the majority of cases, the whole organ is tilted

---

[1] This instrument has been made for me by Messrs. Whicker and Blaise (late Savigny and Co.), of St. James's Street, S.W.

to one side, the os uteri deviating towards the opposite side, so constituting a latero-version. But in one instance, under my care, there remained, three years after discharge of the last abscess, a strong lateral curvature of the body of the uterus, the cervix maintaining its natural position in the vagina. It is to be feared that the setting up of inflammation, and its extension from the uterus to the adjacent tissues, is sometimes attributable to the adoption of heroic methods of local treatment. And this risk demands serious consideration; for there are very few diseases of the female frame which more thoroughly break down the strength and permanently impair or shatter the constitution than pelvic abscess.

Displacement of the adult ovary is a distinct affection from its malposition, as met with in congenital cases, where the organ has been found presenting like a hernia, or occupying one of the labia. It differs also from that deviation of place produced by the gradual drag of uterine displacement, or the pressure of pelvic or abdominal tumours. It was Dr. Rigby who first directed professional attention to this very important variety of ovarian displacement. Previously it had probably been generally classed, like many other affections implicating the female generative cycle, with one or other of the abdominal inflammations; there being, in this case, some resemblance to the symptoms produced during the descent of a renal calculus. When of recent occurrence, displacement or dislocation of the ovary produces a sudden forcing sickening pain, deep seated in the abdomen, and often attended by urgent vomiting and inability to straighten the body. There is a state of anxious depression, almost amounting to collapse, with cold perspirations and a scarcely perceptible pulse. The general symptoms are very similar to those which ensue in the male, when the testicle has been bruised or suddenly strained. The woman cannot bear the least external pressure on the side where the displacement has occurred, and suffers greatly during the internal examination. If the source of this suffering be not recognised, the intensity of the pain ceases after a time, only to recur on any effort or strain, such as the passage of fæces, the movement of flatus in the intestine, on coitus, or any attempt at exertion, or the coming on of that local congestion which precedes menstruation. The direction of the displaced ovary is usually downwards and backwards, so that it comes to lie behind the uterus, and often to occupy the fossa between that organ and the rectum. In one chronic case where the first symptoms occurred two years before the lady came under my care, local examination, whilst the patient lay supine, gave all the indications of retroflexion; for the ovary, lying immediately in the recto-vaginal pouch, resembled both in consistence and shape the retorted fundus uteri.

The diagnosis must be derived from careful attention to the previous history of the case, and from an examination adapted in accordance with the information thus obtained—a rule that should be followed in all disorders of women. The existence of habitual constipation is especially to be noted where the symptoms refer the suffering to the left side. A loaded and distended rectum excites considerable mechanical pressure on the left ovary, tending to force it out of place when powerful purgatives are injudiciously used to drive out the massive contents of the lower bowel. It is unjustifiable, under any circumstances whatever, to administer vehement purgatives to women who have been for a long period " bound up." A very severe case of inflammation of the left ovary came under my notice in 1854, where the symptoms were entirely attributable to the use of strong aperients, in order to remove an accumulation of scybalæ. Rectal examination immediately revealed the real difficulty. Masses of extremely hard feculent matter were removed by means of the handle of a spoon, and the patient had to be supported by powerful stimulants, whilst an immense accumulation, existing above the obstruction, was passed away. The ovarian inflammation and displacement was a matter of subsequent diagnosis and treatment. Such a case illustrates the importance of instituting a rectal examination, wherever the symptoms indicate ovarian mischief, especially of the left side. If the ovary be displaced, without adequate existing mechanical cause to explain its morbid position, the anal examination supplies a valuable auxiliary means of restoring the organ to its position. And in acute cases the use of the double touch—rectal and vaginal—may sometimes afford just as immediate relief from the suffering of ovarian displacement as is experienced when a strangulated hernia is returned.

THE GENERAL TREATMENT to be adopted in treating uterine

displacement depends on a very thorough investigation of the symptoms which have preceded, accompanied, or followed the disorder of uterine place. No two cases ever present precisely the same history, and the exact adaptation of suitable remedies must therefore depend upon precision in the etiological study of each individual case. One has to undo, slowly and cautiously, mischief which has been yet more slowly produced. To accomplish this efficiently, it is necessary to find out where was the commencement of the evil, and to begin from the beginning in order to effect a sound cure. The importance of minute attention to matters which are too often overlooked, as being of trifling import, cannot be too forcibly urged. The arrangement of the female dress has been already alluded to (p. 45), and should be attended to in every case of disorder or disease. The application of powerful local remedial means, mechanical or therapeutical, to an uterus vehemently urged by those vicarious respiratory movements induced whenever the ribs are constricted, is equally irrational and unscientific.

In disorders of place, a well-adjusted belt, steadying the action of the abdominal muscles, is a valuable adjunct in treatment. It should be arranged before the patient moves from her bed; since the stepping quickly to the floor, and the subsequent stirring about the room when she "feels so well," may just undo all the benefit of the night's quiet and sleep. In cases of displacement, the most *absolute local quiet* should be emphatically enjoined to married women while under treatment. In all cases of uterine deviation, there are certain movements which should be especially prohibited, and which may be summed up in a general direction to avoid whatever jerks or jars the body. Rushing quickly downstairs, railway travelling, riding or driving, and exercises which require sudden or impulsive movement, are all done at a risk. On this point patients cannot be too strongly cautioned, for there may thus be undone in a moment the work of days, or even weeks—so long as the uterus retains any impress of the local mischief produced by continued displacement. No exercise is so good as that of quiet walking on a level surface, when due restoration of place has been effected by local means, and its persistence assured by judicious medical treatment, by the tonic influence of rest, of the bath, and of suitable vaginal injections.

Rest.—It must be borne in mind that the advantage gained by long rest in some enjoined position is obtained at the expense of the general health. It is, therefore, far better to adapt some local expedient for support, and permit exercise, than to confine the patient to her couch, at the risk of developing any less tractable disorder, or of the patient becoming a permanent invalid.

The Bath.—The hip-bath is a most important adjunct in the treatment of uterine disorders of place. In the majority of cases it is most conveniently and beneficially used towards noon, instead of early in the morning. The patient should take it as cold as can be borne. A handful of sea salt is often an advantageous addition; or the bath may consist of fresh sea water, if it can be obtained. The amount of reaction is the true test of its usefulness, and of the time for each sitting. Five to fifteen minutes, gradually lengthening the period with those who are feeble, may be taken as representing the average time. If the patient cannot bear a hip-bath for five minutes, she is not arrived at that stage when it is conducive to health.

Suitable vaginal injections, in cases of displacement, are best administered by means of that compact apparatus known as Dr. Kennedy's syphon douche. A multiplicity of instruments have been devised for the same purpose, and it is rather with respect to general convenience that this may be adopted, since the apparatus described by Aetius (A.D. 380—300) for administration of the vaginal injections was just as efficient as the best modern device. In cases of uterine disorder of place, the douche should be used at night; either with cold water, or some simple vegetable astringent, a tannic acid lotion being one of the best. Unless there be leucorrhœal vaginal discharge, or some abnormal and relaxed condition of the mucous membrane, the saline astringents, alum, lead, zinc, &c., are counter-indicated. In such cases they only tend to produce vaginal irritation, if the mucous membrane of the tube is healthy. I have seen cases where casts of the whole length of the vaginal tube were thrown off from the use of saline astringents injudiciously employed.

Careful attention to the symptoms which herald and attend the menstrual periods is very necessary in the treatment of all disorders of place; for it is at those times that the natural renovation of uterine structure is chiefly determined, and the good effects of mechanical restoration of place secured and rendered permanent. In treating of disorders of uterine function and structure, this important influence will come under more immediate consideration.

The method of the medicinal treatment must be arranged in accordance with the particular exigencies of each case. I have already particularly referred to the special value of the hydrochlorate of ammonia, but it may be used in combination either with bichloride of mercury, with sesquichloride of iron, or with the direct alkaline preparations of ammonia, according to the exigencies of individual cases. It is especially important, before thus pursuing a definite course of medicinal treatment, to assure that the digestive organs be in such good order that medicines may be able to exercise their influence. So long as the digestion is disordered, neither food nor physic can duly do their work; and the time spent in setting the stomach to rights, and thus obtaining its valuable co-operation, is certain to be regained, for thereby it is insured that the remedies advised produce the intended therapeutical results. In all chronic cases of Disorder of Uterine Place, the wear of constant pain, the inability to take exercise, the broken sleep, and the deep mental depression, tell upon the digestive powers. In addition to the ordinary symptoms of dyspepsia, there follow those sympathetic headaches which are so intimately connected with functional disorder of some part of the digestive apparatus, either nutritive or eliminative, and are too frequently accredited to the brain itself. The importance of carrying through the inquiry until the original cause of such Headaches is fully determined has been pointed out in my work on this subject.[1]

Where there is disturbance of order in the working of any important system we must consider the functions of every organ, whether digestive or eliminative, the conditions of individual life, the history of foregone disease, whether climacteric, local, or hereditary. Each and all of these must be investigated, and their respective influence considered, before the proper course of medicinal treatment can be satisfactorily determined; and this method of research is especially important before determining to adopt any mode of local treatment of disorders of uterine place.

---

[1] Headaches, their Causes and their Cure. 4th edition.

CHAPTER III.

DISORDERS OF FUNCTION.

THE conditions of healthy pregnancy and natural parturition represent the completed physiological duties of the organs which compose the female generative cycle; the thorough carrying out of that ordained purpose in view of which the correlative endowments of all these organs were arranged. But the functional life of the uterus and its associated organs comprises a very important series of changes, which commonly precede and mark the aptitude for impregnation. Menstruation is the most important of these; the catamenial flux being apparently a subsidiary process in the female economy, established as a means of keeping in repair the organs charged with the duty of continuing the species.

A reasonable explanation of the phenomena and purpose of menstruation has only been practically possible since physiological research demonstrated the changes that take place and the order of their succession. Wanting such precise knowledge, ancient authors fell into evil ways of theorizing; dwelling only on those facts which were best adapted to nourish their particular notions. The menstrual flux in a healthy adult, such as the law recognises by the term " femme sole," occupies about the tenth part of her whole life. A condition so peculiar could not fail to attract attention very early in the history of the race. The first direct reference to the subject (Leviticus, ch. xv. v. 19 *et seq.*) indicates much foregone observation. It had long previously been recognised that at the time of the œstrum, or rut, in animals there was great susceptibility to impregnation (Genesis, ch. xxx.), yet experience taught the lawgiver that in the human female the rule which obtains in animals must be abrogated. And it was probably as a result of the severe injunctions so plainly put in Leviticus (ch. xx. v. 18) that there gradually arose the many curious fancies in reference to the menstrual flux which Pliny[1] notices as received matters of faith in his age, and of which the relics yet survive in the folk-lore of our own time. For in many districts of England it is still believed that a menstruating woman cannot salt meat, make the butter come in the churn, &c. These are but fables, derived originally from Pliny, and disseminated throughout this country in the earliest times of monastic rule. Indeed, one of the most learned of these clerical instructors improved the occasion to enforce a lesson of humility. In his work, "De Naturis Rerum," (*circa* 1200) Alexander Neckam wrote:—

"Nutritur etiam humilitas in homine, si attendat se natum de muliere, quæ sola animal menstruale est, cujus profluvia inter monstrifica merito numerantur. Contactæ his fruges non germinabunt, amittent arbores fœtus, ferrum rubigo corripiet,

---

[1] Nat. History, lib. 7, § 13.

nigrescent æra. Siquid etiam canes inde ederunt, in rabiem efferabuntur, nocituri morsibus, quibus limphaticos faciunt. Bitumen in Judæa, quod Asphaltites lacus gignit, quod separari nequit, apposito cruore illo dissolvitur. Cæterum ipsæ fœminæ, quamdiu sunt in sua lege, non innocentibus oculis contuantur. Aspectu specula vitiant ita ut hebetetur visu fulgor offensus, et solitam æmulationem vultus extinctus splendor amittat faciesque obtusi nitoris quadam caligine nubiletur."

The passage is borrowed almost verbatim from Pliny, but without any acknowledgment. A still earlier monkish authority puts the same matter in another aspect. In the " Oculus Sacerdotum" of Gulielm: de Pagula (pars. 1. cap. 38), the general vileness of humanity is particularly insisted on, and one of the arguments runs thus :—" But observe with what food the embryo is nourished in the uterus ! By the excreted menstrual blood, which ceases from a woman after she has conceived, and is said to be so detestable and foul that after contact with it corn will not germinate, orchards become barren, herbs die, trees shed their fruit. If dogs taste it they are driven to madness."

Faith in these strong assertions has only gradually worn away. So late as the sixteenth century, one who knew well the folk-lore of his time described a kind of leprosy which " doth corrode and eat the flesh to the bones, and the flesh doth rot away," probably lupus exedens, or syphilis, " caused because a child is conceived when the mother is menstruous.

And, therefore, if this infirmity do come by any menstrumous humour, there is no remedy only God and pacience."[1] And in the present time there exists a very general belief, even among educated women, that the troubles, or at best the inconveniences, attending their menstrual periods are entailed by the original wrong of their progenitor ; that, as men father their sins on the old Adam, so women may attribute their sufferings to the original Eve. Judged by modern knowledge, these superstitions have exercised a very beneficial influence. The importance of avoiding sexual congress was authoritatively enjoined ; the women were relieved from toilsome duties during their menstrual times, and if what Pliny wrote at all represents what was then believed, they must have been placed in a sort of social quarantine.

All other parts of the body represent or influence the condition of the individual only. The organs which make up the female generative cycle have to carry out the purpose for which the world was made as it was made. At each menstrual time of a healthful virgin there passes away what might under other conditions have been developed into a new being. The frequent occurrence of these periodic changes among a gregarious race obtains an important significance when considered in relation to the conditions on which we now look back. We recognise the necessity for a regular and progressive increase of

---

[1] The Breviarie of Health : Andrew Boord. He was a shrewd travelling charlatan, and was the first to whom the name of " Merry Andrew " was applied. He latinised his name into Andreas Perforatus.

human life, each generation having its work in the world, as the world ripened, helping to turn to their allotted purpose the hidden stores of creation. All the wood laid down for coal, all the metals hid deep in the earth, all the creatures which continually browsed far beyond their individual necessities (that man might be supplied with flesh for food, and not have to do double digestive duty), all the precious fruit with the wine hidden in its skin, the infusoria building up new shores, whither birds carried seeds to fructify—all these were beneficently provided with creative foreknowledge of the developement of the human race, and of the time when all would come to be turned to account by generations of men; some working with the head, some with the hand. Any other species might have become extinct (as has occurred to those whose work was finished, the great vegetable eaters of the old world); but only a steady and progressive increase of the human race could have assured that series' of successive unveilings of the provident purpose of the Creator which makes up the history of the life of man.

In round numbers, it may be assumed that a healthy woman, living the full span of her life, is so organized that the condition necessary for continuing the race recurs with her nearly four hundred times during the years of her full strength. This condition we designate as menstruation, understanding thereby the periodic evolution of matured ova and the due accomplishment of certain ancillary processes. This provision of power beyond apparent requirements is only in accordance with one of the great laws which obtains throughout the organization. It is conceivable (indeed pathology demonstrates it) that a man living an average life might exist on a considerably diminished supply of organic force: with half-developed muscles, with a vitiated nutritive supply, with only one lung or one kidney, or but half his brain in working order. Such a condition would involve continual effort to preserve vital integrity, and thus the purpose of the being would be rendered subservient to the maintenance of the fabric. Had those physiological changes in the female which are essential for reproduction of the species been similarly restricted, the social results must have been eminently disastrous.

A healthy woman, during the time which we designate as that of uterine life, may be considered capable of bearing, and fulfilling her maternal duties to, twenty successive series of offspring. But at the period of puberty the ovaries are crowded with minute ova, each of them not more than 120th of an inch in diameter. Furthermore, the researches of Dr. Ritchie, of Glasgow, lead to the belief that from very childhood a continuous ovarian evolution occurs, long antecedent to any uterine action or possible impregnation: just as the milk teeth are shed before those which have to do the duty of life come to the surface.[1]

The first stage of a menstrual period comprises those co-

---

[1] "Their numbers are so great, that if only the one-thousandth part of those originally contained in the ovary remain, and no new ones are superadded, there will still be more than sufficient for all the purposes of reproduction."—Dr. Farre.

ordinations, which have for their purpose the evolution of an ovule that has attained maturity. At such a time the relation of the Graafian vesicle to the ovary itself is that of a ripened seed to its containing capsule. Under favourable conditions either might be developed into an independent existence, and, so far as regards the parent, is a foreign body : just as the egg, once cased in its shell, holds no further relations with the parent bird. But the local changes which minister to due evolution of the Graafian vesicle in the virgin, or the ovum in the impregnated female, also subserve other duties. The close sympathy obtaining between the whole series of the generative organs insures co-ordination in the fulfilment of their respective functions, so that each is ready for its share of the work at the appropriate time. With the congestion of the ovarian venous plexus (exercising probably some mechanical influence on the organs themselves), there also ensues a turgescence of the vessels of the Fallopian tubes, inducing erectile action of the fimbriæ and dilatation of the canals, thus ensuring reception of the ovum and free passage in the direction of its appointed course towards the uterus. It is because of this special ovarian congestion that the empty ovisac is found filled with blood when the matured Graafian vesicle or ovum has escaped by dehiscence of the sac wall. This clot, and the membranes of the vacated follicle, speedily undergo degenerative changes, resulting sooner or later in the removal of all traces of their existence. In the virgin the whole process is accomplished with such expedition, that in six or eight weeks only a mere speck distinguishes the place of rupture. The shrivelled capsule is retracted into the substance of the ovary, and by contraction of its cicatrix assists the advancement of the maturing follicle which is to present at the next menstrual ovulation. If the germ be fructified there exists no such occasion for successive development. Then the contained blood clot but very slowly changes, whilst the membrane of the follicle passes gradually into a condition of fatty degeneration. No fresh ova ripen, since the active process of ovulation is suspended during pregnancy, and hence well marked traces of the original habitat of the ovum may be found on the surface of the ovary, even until the birth of the fully developed child; constituting what is known as the true corpus luteum.

The uterus in the inter-menstrual periods presents an exceptional condition of entire functional inactivity. Yet it is eminently essential that this organ shall be constantly in a state of thorough physical aptitude, and the reparation of its tissue efficiently maintained, ready to assume the double duties which pregnancy involves—interstitial developement of uterine substance, and a continuous supply of blood for the fœtus. If we consider menstruation, so far as the uterus itself is concerned, to be a provision for ensuring due renovation of the tissue-substance of the organ, according to the requirements of its work, then those changes which constitute the uterine phenomena of menstruation assume a distinct meaning, and much of the old mystery of the matter is cleared away. Following on the menstrual ovarian dominance, certain well-marked changes ensue in the uterus: the organ becomes congested, and its venous plexus engorged; the cervix is fuller and softer to the touch, and of so deep a tint than an unguarded examination might easily suggest the idea of inflammation. In plethoric women the external organs, the nymphæ, and inner surfaces of the labia, often present that bluish congested appearance commonly seen in pregnancy. Abdominal pressure indicates some tenderness, and where there is any departure, however slight, from the natural state, whether exaggeration of the congestive condition, general hyperæsthesia, or pre-existing local disease, then there occur at each of the menstrual times that suffering which women express by the familiar term of "poorly pains." In the ordinary process of menstruation this local uterine congestion supplies a vital stimulus exactly corresponding to that afforded by local determinations of blood in other parts. There ensue, as demonstrated by Coste, certain increased nutrition changes: the removal of effete tissue and its replacement by new structure—a renewal, in fact, of those parts of the organ which are most important for the due preservation and development of an impregnated ovum. But there is, in addition, an efflux of blood from the uterine cavity. This, I take it, merely represents that provision of supply in excess of demand already referred to as a general physiological law of development. The catamenial flow is certainly an index of the amount of vascular congestion, and its presence indicates a local superabundance of nutritive material. But the occasional occurrence of natural pregnancy, where no such profluvium accompanies ovulation, indicates that the requisite changes effected during menstruation may be fully accomplished without any catamenial flow. Throughout the menstrual life of a healthy woman there is a shedding of blood which amounts altogether to upwards of sixty-eight pounds. It would be opposed to whatever is known of physiology, as well as to the faith that is in us, to suppose that this represents wanton waste of nutritive power. It seems probable that the purpose of the increased uterine congestion is to ensure that there shall be ready an ample supply of blood to initiate the growth of a fertilised germ; so that the ancient idea of the catamenial flow being provided for nourishment of the fœtus, might be considered as expressing a right theory in wrong terms.

As the process of menstruation draws to its close, the discharge becomes paler, and in health its cessation is gradual, the blood corpuscles becoming rare and epithelium more abundant; for the parts external to the uterus share, throughout, the exalted physiological action attending menstruation. The natural secretion of the mucous membranes of the passage is therefore increased; and its prolonged continuance after a period has ceased forms the early history of many cases of vaginal leucorrhœa.

The process of menstruation is a distinctly physical endowment. However modified by external circumstances, there is still an original uniform type with which these variations may be compared. That marvellous adaptability (special to the human race) by means of which life can be healthily maintained under the most diverse conditions, involves very considerable modifications of organization or function, in accordance with the changes of climate or mode of existence. Between savage and civilised life in the same country there may exist just as great variations of physical condition as obtain between the inhabitants of India and Iceland; and the influences thus exercised, whether climacteric or social, affect in a marked degree the order of uterine function. Thus, in this country, many bathing women continue their avocation throughout the menstrual times without inconvenience, and gipsies pursue their tramp immediately after parturition. But in delicately nurtured women most disastrous results ensue if they are accidentally exposed to similar conditions.

For due consideration of the original functional co-relations, we must go back, as nearly as may be, to that state of life which obtained before any artificial restraints, variations of climate, or exigencies of existence, compelled a departure from the pristine order. Thus reverting to the original intent of the menstrual function, its first occurrence may be assumed to represent a condition of ripeness in the system for the work of reproduction. This is nearly the order of development which still obtains in those warmer climates which cradled the human race. There it is still observed that the physical changes which accompany puberty are developed to an extent not witnessed in a more artificial condition of life and a less genial climate. But the co-relations of the uterine functions remain unaltered among the natives of the coldest countries, so long as life is carried on just in accordance with the exigencies of the climate. The Syrian woman is nubile years before the Esquimaux, yet the relation of fecundity to the first occurrence of menstruation presents very slight variation. The time of puberty has in reality been judged by an artificial standard; not according to the conditions which determine development of womanhood under different climates and phases of social life, but always with relation to certain statistical results. If one girl first menstruates at twelve and another at eighteen, it is eminently important to ascertain, if it be possible, why this variation occurs, and to distinguish whether it is right to look on this wide difference as natural or abnormal.

The intermediate climates of the world include those in which civilization has been most highly developed and the race rendered most independent of external conditions. Warm clothing, heated rooms, stimulating diets, sedentary habits, intellectual cultivation, and other influences which quicken functional development, are just those which retard the naturally coincident condition of redundant physical vigour requisite for the due nurture of the germ, the growth of the fœtus, and the sustenance of the child. Under such artificial conditions of life, it became a social necessity that some separation should be made between the time of puberty and that which acknowledges a fitness for child-bearing. The history of woman's life in different climates of the world exhibits a tacit acknowledgment of this variation, and the experience of every-day practice affords evidence of its importance. Thus, for example, in females of strumous habit (and scrofula is especially a disease of artificial culture) the first menstrual period usually occurs early in life; but it is prudent, on account of the defective state of physical nutrition, to delay marriage until the frame has attained its mature development and its utmost strength.

Such an enforced separation between the first occurrence of menstruation and the nubile period implies a great variation in the order of menstrual life at its commencement. Under artificial conditions of existence the duties of the generative cycle are so modified that the first few years of menstruation are merely preparative; the local changes being natural, the general development inefficient. Those very conditions of social life which have gradually effected a wide separation between the pubescent and nubile periods also exercise an important influence in retarding or accelerating the changes of puberty. Here prematurity is of far more serious import than delayed menstruation; for it is when local functional change is greatly in advance of physical development that there especially ensue early manifestations of constitutional disease, or evidences of such exhaustive effort that the period of puberty becomes one of anxiety.

The irregularities which accompany the establishment of menstruation range through so wide an area that it is rare to find two cases in which all the conditions are identical. For every point in the young life must be taken into account—the hereditary influence, the progress of early diseases, the growth and dental development, the diet, and the mode of mental and physical education. It is only by very careful research that the aberrations which accompany the first development of the menstrual function can be accurately understood, and the means proper for insuring fulfilment of the Order of Function adopted.

It is the general rather than the functional health which in the majority of cases has to be regarded; bearing in mind that the periodic maturation of a developed Graafian vesicle is the earliest change of menstruation, that the condition of the general health governs and modifies this primary change, and that the condition of the uterus, its congestion, development, and catamenial efflux, should, at this period of life, only assume a secondary importance.

At the other extreme of active uterine life the same disordered relations very frequently occur between the functions of the generative cycle and the constitutional condition. In a primitive state, with the appointed physiological sequence accurately followed, the cessation of menstruation was probably coincident with that great climacteric change which marks a readjustment of the relations of nutrition in accordance with the decline of life, and of those conditions " which should accompany old age." But in a very considerable number of women living ordinary lives, these changes are by no means coincident. In some, especially those who have a tendency to obesity and pursue a tranquil existence, the catamenia may cease, slowly and naturally, in middle life, without any inconvenience attending the change; but the symptoms which mark the climacteric period may not ensue for ten or twelve years subsequently. The reverse order chiefly obtains with women who have undergone numerous miscarriages or borne children very rapidly. At a comparatively early age they pass into premature decrepitude without suffering and without disease. They grow old before their time, and the change is often very sudden; the hair becomes gray, the features sharpen, and wrinkles fold themselves in the skin, the limbs lose their roundness, and exercise is only a synonym for exertion. Yet the catamenial periods may go on with their wonted regularity, and only cease at the natural time; if age is to be reckoned by years of life.

The influences which determine the periodic return of the menstrual condition are but imperfectly understood, although it has been a fertile ground of speculation since the earliest times. Anciently it was generally believed that the phases of the moon influenced the menstrual molimen; and among the Chinese the periodic flux of a woman is still called her "moons." The general condition of nutrition importantly influences the occurrence and modifies the extent and regularity of menstruation, and beyond this general statement it is not safe to venture. Thus in cases of sudden and severe illness, in the progress of exhaustive disease, and during the first months of convalescence, menstruation is commonly arrested; but the recorded exceptions are numerous. I have in several cases known the periods to recur naturally and regularly in advanced phthisis, and, in one instance, menstruation ensued on the day preceding the patient's death: in another case the menstrual flux appeared on the very day of an eruption of small-pox. However obscured and tangled are the causes which determine the monthly recurrence, their existence is certain, and waits a scientific explanation; for the only effect of attributing the changes to the laws of periodicity about which so much has been written, is to check the progress of healthy research. It would be just as reasonable for one standing near an overshot water-wheel, and timing its revolution watch in hand, to credit the regularity of the movement to inherent periodicity; taking no note of the influence of the stream above in filling the buckets of the wheel.

AMENORRHŒA includes generally all those cases where menstruation is deficient. But the term is applied to widely differing conditions; from simple defect in regularity, quantity, or quality, to an entire absence of the catamenia, which may be either original (*emansio mensium*), acquired (*suppressio mensium*), or so associated with marked and peculiar constitutional changes that the word Chlorosis has been adapted to signify a generally unhealthy state, in which many things are wrong in addition to the menstrual deficiency. The word amenorrhœa is therefore only a convenient term, under which are grouped a series of very diverse conditions, and may be understood to express a certain deficient fulfilment of menstrual function so marked that it can be adopted as a starting-point from which the investigation of the history of each case may commence, the causes of the disorder be traced to their source, and the treatment proportionally modified and adapted. The difficulty begins where the definition ends.

In describing the phenomena of healthy menstruation, these have been arranged in a certain order, comprising three distinct influences: systemic, ovarian, and uterine. This plan of the order of healthy functional change at once acquires a practical bearing if it assist the diagnosis by enabling the practitioner to detect where the defect in regularity has its origin, and to select his remedies accordingly.

Certain medicines have, by long usage, come to be credited with specific influence in determining the occurrence of menstruation. This reputation has caused them to be grouped together as Emmenagogues (ἐμμήνια the menstrual discharge, ἀγωγὸς an eliciting or evoking). It is evident that if the natural process of menstruation comprise the successive stages already described, an indiscriminate use of the medicines included in the long catalogue of emmenagogues must present very marked discrepancies in the result. This variation of action, in reality, exceeds that of any other class of remedies, and the irregularity and apparently inexplicable difference has again and again been made the subject of special comment. Remedies reputed as successful by one practitioner, utterly fail when tested by other observers; and the long list of drugs, in turn recommended and rejected, indicates that the elements which governed the success or failure have been imperfectly understood. In every case of amenorrhœa it is essential that the investigation should be pursued until the cause that determines the deficiency is detected. But in many cases a difficulty arises at the very outset of the inquiry, when it is necessary to distinguish between the original causes of the disordered menstruation and the general symptoms that have preceded or accompanied the arrest of functional action, often the direct results of the same untoward condition that caused the arrest of menstruation.

1. *Systemic Amenorrhœa.*—Scanty, delayed, or arrested menstruation depending on constitutional causes, includes a wide range of cases. It may be that the circulatory system is at fault, as in pale, anæmic, overgrown girls; or the nervous system, as in sluggish, inanimate patients. It may be that the nutrition of the body is depraved by bad food taken, by good food ill-digested, or by retention within the body of excrementitious matter, either in the loaded intestines, or by reason of insufficient depuration, whether by the liver, kidneys, or other excretive organ. There may be some hereditary constitutional taint, or some influence from without which modifies the general health. Cases occur in this country where menstruation ensues regularly during the summer months, and is partially or entirely absent during winter; removal to a warm climate being followed by a natural establishment of the function.

It very commonly happens that healthy country-girls, coming to reside in London, suffer from amenorrhœa. This is especially frequent with servants and work-girls, and constitutes a form of amenorrhœa which it would be eminently injudicious to treat by any of those methods which exercise a direct stimulative influence on the generative organs. But the most illustrative cases of systemic amenorrhœa occur in women convalescent from diseases of an exhaustive kind. Very frequently several periods pass without fully restoring menstruation, though the recurrence of a distinct effort may be detected; at each time increasing, as the strength is regained, until the healthy relief is fully established. The meaning of this arrest is evident. Regular ovulation, and with the attendant menstrual changes, would possibly involve an urgent and immediate call for a nutritive supply to sustain the germ. The system, being itself under repair, cannot afford this; the demand could only be met at the risk of permanent injury, and so the primary and essential process of menstruation is deferred. Those exceptional cases in which pregnancy ensues before a woman's strength is restored after an illness, are almost invariably attended with unusual suffering, and often followed by very serious results.

A considerable number of the remedies successfully employed in amenorrhœa effect their purpose by improving the general health; they have, in fact, no direct influence whatever on the generative cycle in women, other than that which they exert over all the organs and functions of the body, equally in males and females; and as the majority of cases of amenorrhœa recognise a systemic origin, the comparatively great success of constitutional treatment is readily understood. The various preparations of iron and of strychnia, of iodine, of the mineral acids and vegetable bitters; the influence of pure air, good food, and of bathing; the providing that due nutriment shall be supplied and excrementitious matter freely eliminated—all these are of acknowledged value in restoring healthy menstruation, but exercise no specific local influence.

Of the preparations of iron, the sesquioxide and compound iron pill, long favourite remedies in cases of amenorrhœa, are now banished from the pharmacopœia, and the mistura ferri co., or Griffiths' mixture, another unstable preparation, might also be beneficially superseded by the more elegant and certain compounds which modern pharmacy has added to our resources. Among these may be especially mentioned the citrate and tartrate and acetate, the saccharated carbonate, the scaled pyrophosphate, syrup of the iodide and of the phosphate, and the sulphate, saccharated or granulated in order to prevent oxydation. The new tincture of perchloride of iron (P.B.) is, according to my experience, a less valuable preparation than the old muriated tincture, which contained a proportion of hydrochloric ether. It is in amenorrhœa with marked anæmia that iron is especially indicated. Where the want of vigour and of general tone is obviously traceable to the nervous system, the preparations of strychnia often prove very beneficial. This drug was first recommended as an emmenagogue by Sir T. Baddeley. It has undergone the usual fate, necessarily failing where employed in unsuitable cases. I have for some years almost exclusively employed in asthenic amenorrhœa (as well as in many other cases) the ignatia amara in place of the nux vomica. I believe it less liable to produce those excitant influences occasionally occurring, even when the dose of strychnia has been very minute.

The vegetable bitters and the mineral acids often act as emmenagogues, in so far that they ensure a proper order of the food-changes; thus affording healthy nourishment, and inducing due fulfilment of functional action. But this series of processes would be of little avail were the blood itself already loaded with noxious elements. If the air breathed be deficient in oxygen or otherwise vitiated, this implies a partial arrest in the ultimate assimilation of the nutritive material prepared with such elaborate care. Just as retention of urea from inefficient renal action poisons the blood, so accumulated fæces may produce by resorption a toxæmic influence quite as marked as in cases where there is excess of bile in the blood from hepatic obstruction. The injurious influence of defective sewerage external to the body, has deservedly attracted great attention of late years. But the poison is the same, whether generated within or breathed in foul air from without. In all such cases, many stages intervene between the state of health and the time when the resistant powers of the frame succumb to the noxious influence, give up the fight, and allow full sweep to the poison. For every one laid up with typhoid fever, there are hundreds exposed to the same influences who manage to hold their own, and, though notably reduced or constitutionally damaged and enfeebled, escape actual prostration by fever. In women exposed to such noxious influences, the amenorrhœa is only one of many evidences of toxæmia.

It is especially among the poor of large cities that such cases are met with, and they very constantly refer their general symptoms to the arrest of menstruation. In such cases, pure air and depurative remedies, especially combinations of chlorine, may act as emmenagogues.

There are certain cases of amenorrhœa of systemic origin, in which all ordinary remedies fail, but where arsenic exercises a marked beneficial effect, the menstruation recurring so soon as the system presents indications of the influence of the drug. There is neither a plethoric state, the sthenic amenorrhœa of some observers, nor is there an anæmic or asthenic condition. But the cases usually present some approach to that unhealthy state of the skin which in an extreme degree marks diseases where arsenic usually acts as a specific. In several such cases where the skin was dry and hard, or scurfy, arsenic has succeeded in my own practice, when a long succession of other remedies had previously failed to induce or re-establish menstruation.

2. *Amenorrhœa due to some defective action in the ovaries or the uterus.*—The evidence in such cases is both negative and positive. There is the absence of those general characteristics already mentioned, and the symptoms follow " certain periods more or less well marked in the regularity of their return, when a special disorder of the nervous and vascular systems, and various forms of local suffering referred more or less distinctly to the womb or to the parts adjacent, announce a sort of imperfect menstrual effort." [1] Where the deficient menstrua-

---

[1] Dr. West: Diseases of Women, p. 37.

tion is due to some constitutional cause, the symptoms are equally well marked at all times. Where amenorrhœa depends on ineffective action of the ovaries or uterus, there is usually present some considerable periodic exacerbation. Where long intervals elapse between catamenial periods, the local cause is, I believe, usually ovarian; where the amount of relief is deficient, the flow appearing only for a few hours, or presenting an appearance scarcely different from the leucorrhœa which commonly accompanies such cases, then I believe the uterus is generally at fault.

In cases where the local changes are not on a par with the state of the general health, there is often a notable deficiency of developement throughout the whole system of organs connected with the generative function. The mammæ are small, and if an internal examination be necessary, the uterus is found to be diminutive, often retaining in a greater or less degree that curvature forwards already described (p. 64). I believe that in the large majority of cases where amenorrhœa occurs in robust girls, and is chiefly marked by general symptoms of plethora, the derangement is of local origin. Where the cause of the amenorrhœa is systemic, the treatment should be continued perseveringly; where the symptoms indicate a local cause, attention should be especially directed to the time when the menstrual period would be due.

Those ovarian changes which form the essential part of menstruation may fail in two ways: either by deficiency of natural development of the organs, or an excessive irritability equal to that of dysmenorrhœa, but without the accruing relief. It is in the former class of cases that the numerous methods which act exclusively by direct sympathetic excitation, produce an emmenagogue influence—stimulant liniments to the loins, hot poultices, dry cupping to the breasts, assafœtida and turpentine enemata, &c., and the application of ice as advised by Dr. Chapman.

The numerous cases in which electricity has been successfully employed for the relief of amenorrhœa undoubtedly owe their good result to the local influence of this agency; but it is important to discriminate between the purposes which different currents subserve. As ordinarily employed the results obtained might be due either to direct uterine stimulus, or to a similar influence on the ovaries. By that method of using electricity which owes its origin to Faraday, which has been physiologically investigated by Duchenne, and which can be so readily applied with the neat apparatus devised by Messrs. Legendre and Morin,[1] it is easy to regulate the character of the current, influencing either the motor or sensory nerves at will. It is by the latter or secondary current that the ovaries are affected, the poles being applied to the loin and groin. Where an irritable state of one or both ovaries impedes the healthy menstrual action, it constitutes the second form of amenorrhœa of ovarian origin. There is always some local tenderness and pain on exertion, and the condition nearly corresponds to that state of irritability which interferes with the

---

[1] Appareil pour Faradisation. It may be procured from Messrs. Wheeler and Blaire, 67, St. James's-street.

due discharge of their proper functions in many organs—notably the liver, stomach, and bladder. It is here that sedatives, especially aconite and Indian hemp, prove beneficial, and that bromide of potassium, taken internally, and counter-irritants applied over the ovarian region, have been found to relieve the suffering, and restore the natural function.

Amenorrhœa attributable to the uterus may be due to some original organic defect, to deficiency of development of the organ, to the results of foregone disease of its tissues, or to occlusion of the cervix. The following remarkable case illustrates the first condition :—

A. E., æt. 19, single, of middle height, regular and delicate features, figure well developed and proportioned, luxuriant brown hair, perfect teeth, a soft, womanly voice, the bosoms round, and skin soft and smooth, applied to me in 1853, for relief of occasional severe attacks of tic-douloureux. On inquiry I learnt from her mother that the menstruation was regular, but very slight, "in fact, a mere show," which had first appeared at the age of fifteen. The patient being cured of her neuralgia, after a few visits, did not again come under notice for nearly two years. Then her mother requested a visit, and explained that there had been some difficulty in the consummation of marriage. I supposed it would prove one of the ordinary cases which arise under these circumstances. But on examination I found that the vagina ended in a cul-de-sac about an inch and a half from the vulva, and such had been the arrest of uterine development, that rectal examination only detected a rudimentary organ of the size of a large pea. The ovaries were recognised as healthy both in size and position. It is evident that in this case the ovarian influence had specially determined some vaginal discharge at the menstrual periods, but that no true catamenia occurred. The mother had attributed the deficiency to general want of healthy tone; and the physical development of the patient was so womanly, that nothing but local examination would have determined the existence of such an exceptional organic deficiency.

Occlusion of the uterine orifice may be partial or complete. That menstruation should under the latter condition persistently recur with, so far as can be judged, a due catamenial efflux from the walls of the uterus, indicates the potential influence of the systemic and ovarian changes in the causation of menstruation. The tar-like fluid evacuated when an occluded uterus has been opened, shows the extent to which resorption of the watery part of the menstrual blood had occurred previously; but there occasionally present cases where it would seem that some spasmodic closure of the internal os of the cervix, or possibly of its whole canal is induced; where due symptoms of menstruation occur in their accustomed order, and there follows, after a certain delay, either the expulsion of blood clots, or a free efflux of the uterine contents, at regular intervals.

The uterus was formerly accredited as the chief agent of menstruation. Hence the employment for amenorrhœa of means known to specifically influence the organ. The list of emmenagogues comprises a large number which only act through their direct uterine influence, but must be mischievous in cases where the amenorrhœa is due to other causes. Among these immediate uterine stimulants may be mentioned Sir J. Y. Simpson's galvanic pessaries, and his method of mechanical irrritation by sucking into the holes of an exhausted tube different parts of the intra-uterine mucous membrane. For such cases the introduction of intra-uterine bougies, the use of ammonia injections, and the administration of cantharides, savine, and large doses of aloes, have been advised; but their employment needs very nice discrimination, for such decided means may only be used when the diagnosis of the uterine origin of amenorrhœa is clearly established. In any other cases, only mischief could result from the employment of means specially adapted to produce distinct local influence. Among the numerous emmenagogue remedies which have been alternately praised and contemned, the ergot of rye occupies an important place. When menstruation was considered as the fulfilment of an uterine function, the ordinary operation of ergot evidently suggested its employment as a deobstruent. That it failed generally, and occasionally succeeded where all other means had been tried in vain, was just the result to be anticipated from its indiscriminate use as an emmenagogue. The uncertainty of the preparations formerly used might also have had something to do with the frequent failure of the drug. After considerable experience in the employment of ergot as an emmenagogue, in cases where the causes of the amenorrhœa is uterine, I believe its efficacy to be indubitable; but it is scarcely necessary to add that the greatest caution should be exercised, and that the drug should never be used if there be the least reason to suspect some cause of functional deficiency which the patient may omit to mention.

The best preparations are the powder, infusion, and liquid extract. The following cases all presented indications for its use :—

J. M., æt. 21. Amenorrhœa three months, following an attack of menorrhagia caused by being suddenly frightened just when her menses were due. Ordered twenty drops of the liquid extract twice a day. The catamenia appeared on the third day.

E. W., æt. 32. Caught a severe cold while menstruating. Catamenia ceased suddenly, with severe pain and tenderness in the uterine region and headaches; two periods have elapsed without any show. Ordered pulv. ergot. gr. viij. once a day. Menses reappeared after six doses.

M. L., æt. 21. Strong healthy-looking girl, regular till six months ago, when a large abscess formed in axilla. Has intense frontal headache at each period, with a forcing sensation in the body, but no menstrual show. The ergot was given twice a day. Menstruation occurred after it had been taken for a week.

C. B., æt. 37. Suffers from vomiting and extreme prostration, consequent on the small amount of food she can retain. Dates her suffering to a menstrual check three months ago. Had had severe "body pains" at each time, but no show. Menstruation occurred for one day after taking four doses of the liquid extract, with immediate relief to the sickness. The next ensuing period passed naturally without taking any medicine.

A. L., æt. 33. Has had deficient menstrual flow since puberty; menses rarely lasting more than one day; always with much pain in body and legs. For last six months (in winter) have ceased altogether. Took powdered ergot for three days, when the catamenia appeared. The drug was again resorted to four days prior to the next two periods, when the menstruation occurred with but little pain, lasting three days each time. Subsequently married and became pregnant.

C. C., æt. 15. Has severe hysterical fits, occurring twice or oftener each day, and becoming more convulsive, with much struggling. These have continued for upwards of a year, with the exception of three months in the summer, when the menses appeared regularly and healthily. She indicates the seat of the first sensation of an impending fit by placing her hand on the uterine region. Ordered ergot and magnes. sulph. twice a day. The fits ceased entirely on the third, and menstruation ensued on the eighth day; a fit of three hours' duration preceding the appearance. The catamenia were subsequently regular, the health being improved by quinine and iron.

These cases are selected from a number so great as to indubitably prove that the ergot of rye does exercise a specific influence, either direct or transmitted, and that in appropriate cases it may be confidently employed; and they further indicate the necessity for carefully searching out the origin of the menstrual disorder through all the heterogeneous symptoms which so frequently complicate the history. But it is essential to bear in mind that nothing can justify the use of any emmenagogue exercising a specific local influence if there be the shadow of a doubt as to the presence of pregnancy.

Suppression of Menstruation means an arrest of the process in mid-way, and when all things were ready for the immediate production of the catamenial flux, or for its maintenance during the natural time. It therefore differs materially from absent or delayed menstruation. Suppression may occur at any age or under any conditions of life between the periods of puberty and change. It is usually due to external causes, which may be traced either to powerful mental influence or to some physical check without direct implication of the generative organs. There is an important practical difference in the results which ensue.

Mental Influence producing Suppression.—Sudden shocks or fright, entirely irrespective of any physical influence, may produce an immediate arrest of the menstrual flow, just as the same causes will stop the whole process of digestion. Many months may elapse before the patient again exhibits any symptoms indicating a return of menstruation; and if the age approach to that time when the function should naturally cease, there may be no renewal of the effort.

I, select twelve cases in which menstruation had been healthily performed up to the date of its sudden suppression from the causes noted; all occurring during the catamenial period :—

1. æt. 17. Frightened by burglars.
2. æt. 19. Assaulted by a drunken man.
3. æt. 20. Struck by lightning.
4. æt. 24. Attacked by a dog.
5. æt. 26. Frightened by a snake.
6. æt. 21. Found the fellow-servant with whom she slept was dead by her side.
7. æt. 38. Opened the house-door when her husband was brought home dead.
8. æt. 30. Alarmed by sudden death of a child.
9. æt. 22. Ditto, ditto, of a brother.
10. æt. 27. Frightened by dress catching fire.

11. æt. 33. Husband died suddenly from bursting of an aneurism.
12. æt. 25. Agitated by witnessing the capsize of a boat with some near relatives on board.

In only two of these cases could any notable physical results be traced. In the first, there was chorea; in the third, hemiplegia from the stroke of lightning. In all, there was immediate check of menstruation. In cases seven, eight, and eleven, it did not recur again, so far as I could trace the cases. In the other nine it reappeared after the lapse of more or less time. Where suppression is exclusively due to mental impression, there do not usually ensue those marked symptoms which occur when the arrest has ensued from some physical shock; and I have been led to consider these cases as approximating in character to that form of amenorrhœa in which there is deficiency of the vital stimulus which determines or governs the process of ovarian functional changes, with which a catamenial period begins.

Where suppression is due to physical causes the results which ensue may, on the other hand, be very severe, may lay the foundation of subsequent local disease, or produce very grave and peculiar general results. The most common of all physical causes is sudden exposure to cold and wet; especially if the general health be at the time enfeebled. Young girls, not properly warned, and frightened at the first appearance of menstruation, sometimes, in their ignorance, use cold applications to stop the flow, and thus induce sudden suppression and subsequent chlorosis. Other cases have come under observation, where the appearance of the catamenial flux on the eve of a party, or other engagement, has been purposely and deliberately checked by women whose experience should have taught them better. But the most frequent cases of suppression are those in which some accident or uncontrollable impulse has unintentionally induced the sudden check. At p. 124 I have given some cases of this nature. The injurious influence produced by menstrual suppression is in an inverse ratio to the susceptibility to its occurrence. Some women are so sensitively organized, that dipping the hands into cold water, or the moving out of a warm bed, will suffice to check, or entirely arrest, the menstrual flow, without any notable after-symptoms ensuing. Others can endure exposure, and even great fatigue, during menstruation, without the flux being affected; but it is in this latter class, where some vehement effort or extreme exposure has suddenly deranged the functional order, that the most severe sequences of menstrual suppression ensue. The ill results which arise from such sudden suppression may follow directly, or be only gradually developed. The effects may be either local or general.

Sudden and severe local suffering, whether ovarian or uterine, occurring in a previously healthy woman, should always induce careful inquiries as to any menstrual check. The nature of the cause (if this be exposure to cold or damp), as well as the character of the suffering, might easily mislead. The disease is grouped under that comprehensive term, "inflammation of the bowels," and the local mischief, whether oophritis or uterine congestion, escapes attention. In such cases, or where women neglect to obtain proper professional advice, dysmenorrhœa usually ensues at succeeding periods. But sudden arrest of menstruation may, although rarely, lead to the occurrence of true pelvi-peritonitis, apparently by direct extension; or the flow may take an untoward direction, producing an effusion of blood either into the cavity of the pelvis (intra-peritoneal hæmatocele) or among the meshes of connective structure (peri-uterine hæmatocele). In these cases early diagnosis is of the utmost importance; for by active treatment absorption of the blood is possible, and the occurrence of pelvic abscess may be averted. But when this serious result has ensued, whether consequent on menstrual suppression or parturition, it often happens that after the first evacuation of the matter, the local determination of blood attending each catamenial period induces reaccumulation and discharge of pus at those times during many subsequent months. In all cases of menstrual suppression, accompanied by local symptoms, it is absolutely essential that a careful vaginal examination be instituted without delay. Where the suppression is sudden, and obviously due to physical causes, although there be an entire absence of local symptoms, very serious general results may ensue. The most marked illustrations are seen in cases where the injurious influence is exercised through the nervous system. Dr. Pritchard writes, that "sudden suppressions of the catamenia are frequently followed by diseases of the nervous system of various kinds. Females exposed to cold experience a suppression of the catamenia, followed, in some instances, immediately by fits of epilepsy or hysteria, the attacks of which are so sudden as to illustrate the connexion of cause and effect." Esquirol says, " Among women of all classes menstruation, either because it has been with difficulty established, or has been suppressed, or in consequence of its final suppression, is one of the most common causes of mania." Dr. Duckworth Williams has cited a number of instances illustrating the same view. The following case occurred in my own practice :—

Lady ——, æt. 23, married, no family, healthy and regular until March, 1863. Tempted by the bright sun, she left her close carriage in order to walk home, on the second day of a more than usually profuse catamenial period. Turning the corner of a street near her residence she met a cold sharp east wind, which " chilled her whole frame." On entering the drawing-room she deliberately walked to the fire and sat down on it. Luckily, her dress was velvet and not very inflammable, and a footman was in the room. She was carried upstairs and had a vehement hysterical attack. By the aid of stimulants and warm local applications, she recovered in a short time, and the menses, which had been suddenly arrested, recurred after a few doses of nitric ether and henbane. This lady described herself as feeling that her consciousness could only be retained by a great effort from the time that she felt the sudden chill of the cold wind ; that, on entering the warm room she had a dim sense of extreme personal cold, and of the fire as a something which would afford heat ; she recollected nothing more of what passed during several subsequent hours.

A sudden suppression of the menstrual secretion sometimes influences the establishment of disease in parts having no immediate relation with the generative cycle. Thus inflammation of the lungs or pleuræ, jaundice, cardiac disease, and many acute affections, dropsy, renal congestion (nearly approaching to true nephritis), have often been noted as coincident with menstrual suppression. It is evident that these diseases may have owed their origin to the same causes which determined the catamenial check. Still, knowing that sudden arrest of the menstrual secretion may produce very powerful influences on distant and diverse organs, and that defect of catamenial relief is frequently the only recognisable preliminary to those remarkable blood-changes which occur in chlorosis, it is of obvious importance in all cases of acute diseases in women, to ascertain with the utmost precision, whether any disturbance of the order of menstruation has preceded or accompanied the first development of the symptoms.

Taking the general range of cases which in daily practice fall under notice, it is comparatively seldom that we meet with instances of acute disease which present to the full all the characteristic symptoms, or follow precisely the order, described in books. But, every day there fall under notice cases, in which a knowledge of the definitions and descriptions of disease guides us to its recognition in a less developed stage. The "touch of pleurisy," the "threatening of gout," the "petit mal" of epilepsy, the ischuria of lithiasis, &c., hold an evident kinship with well-known diseases; and require that this be acknowledged both in diagnosis and treatment. In the same way there may occur partial or imperfect manifestations of those disorders of function here included under the general title of amenorrhœa; accompanied by symptoms which require to be very carefully investigated lest their original cause be missed. Sudden and total suppression of the catamenia is a matter which at once arrests attention, but cases constantly occur in practice where the menstrual efflux is stated to be regular, yet a little inquiry elicits that there has been considerable foregone irregularity; that the intervals have been abnormally long, or that the amount of relief is disproportionate to the prodromata ushering in the sanguineous discharge. Nor is it unfrequent to meet with cases where this suffering is in itself considered sufficient to justify a belief that all is as it should be. In some there is little more than a temporary leucorrhœa, or the efflux continues but a very few hours. If *absolute* amenorrhœa, whatever its cause, be attended with certain well-marked results, it is only in accordance with general knowledge and experience that a *partial* disorder of the menstrual function should induce a series of less distinctive symptoms; which, however, can only be adequately treated by precognition of the original defect in functional activity.

But there is one group of symptoms, determined by arrest or inefficient performance of the menstrual function, which may claim special consideration, since it is either omitted or only lightly alluded to in the standard works on uterine disorders. So numerous and so distinctive are those cases which have occurred in my own practice as to justify the belief that this characteristic form of suffering is a very frequent, as it is a very painful, accompaniment of deficient menstruation.

My attention was especially directed to this point by three nearly coincident cases. The patients were unmarried, aged respectively 17, 21, and 24, of good social position, and free from any hereditary taint. There was defective menstruation: in one, total arrest; in another, dysmenorrhœa, with but little relief; in the third, a mere show, lasting but a few hours. My services were required because of severe pains in the large joints, especially the knees and ankles, which, in two of the cases, absolutely precluded the least movement. There was a history of "rheumatic fever" having occurred some time previously (respectively one year, two years, and eight months) before I saw the patients; and each case had been thus diagnosed and treated by the professional attendants. But attentive examination of the heart-sounds afforded only negative results; there being no evidence whatever of any valvular or pericardial lesion. On further inquiry it was elicited that the previous attacks had been preceded by some foregone derangement of the menstrual function, more or less resembling the condition present when the patients came under my notice.

The relation between disordered uterine function and the occurrence of severe joint-pains arrested the attention of the late Dr. Todd, who remarks, "The connexion between rheumatic fever and deranged uterine secretions is very remarkable. Some of the most severe cases I have ever seen have followed dysmenorrhœa."[1] The frequent concurrence of dysmenorrhœa with inefficient menstrual flux must be remembered; since Dr. Todd refers to something beyond mere painful menstruation, where symptoms akin to rheumatism do not occur. In a hundred cases of amenorrhœa characterized by marked deficiency in amount, by irregularity of occurrence, or by absolute menstrual arrest, I found that, in 72, pains in the joints, especially in the knees and ankles, were mentioned among the chief causes of suffering. I excepted from the list all cases where there was evidence of hereditary disease; or where the heart presented indications of organic complication from foregone acute rheumatism. In some of these patients the pain and tenderness were as great as in true rheumatism; but in none of them was there that increase of local temperature which accompanies the general disease. Moreover, although there was, in the most severe cases, considerable swelling, this appeared to ensue some days subsequent to the commencement of suffering. The amount of this pain varied both in extent and location, sometimes absolutely hindering all movement, sometimes only inducing a stiffness and aching sensation in the affected joints. In no cases that I have seen was there that profuse general perspiration which accompanies acute rheumatism.

The importance of recognising such a connexion between

---

[1] Clinical Lectures on certain Acute Diseases.

defective menstrual relief and an accession of local pains nearly resembling rheumatism is obvious. Applications to the painful parts, or treatment directed exclusively for the relief of the supposed rheumatic seizure, would only exercise a palliative influence; restoration or establishment of the natural menstrual relief being the method obviously indicated for insuring permanent benefit.

If retention within the system of products which, in health, would be eliminated at the menstrual periods, induces certain grave and well-marked results, it is evident that the extent of these results must be influenced by the state of individual health of the patient. It is important to give due credit, but not more than is due, to the causes in operation. Though amenorrhœa occur, there may also co-exist serious disease, which is entirely independent of the functional arrest. The error that may hence arise is well illustrated in the published correspondence of the famous Dr. Fothergill, where it is mentioned, as an ordinary pathological sequence, that a patient is judged to be "labouring under many of the symptoms of a beginning phthisis from an obstruction of the menses." True Chlorosis represents a condition where the blood is materially deteriorated; its proximate cause being some defect or arrest of the natural menstrual efflux. External circumstances greatly modify the extent to which this influence operates; and there is much truth in the observation of Dr. Lettsom, that "sentiments respecting the delicacy of the sex constitute an apology for inducing a delicacy of constitution, as if frailty were a favourable acquisition, and bodily imbecility the source of mental happiness."[1]

If such marked results frequently occur among young women so cherished and guarded that real hardship is unknown to them, it is to be remembered that the same cause is in operation among the poor; where deficient food, foul air, sedentary occupations, and scanty clothing afford vantage-ground for rapid advance of disease. And medical statistics are principally gathered from the poor. It is matter for consideration, whether in such cases poisonous influences generated from within, may not produce just as formidable results as those received from without. In the well-nurtured girl simple Chlorosis may follow deficient menstruation; in the half-starved work-girl there may ensue fever of that character distinctly due to blood-empoisonments and attributed to some cause (as the foul air of an open sewer) acting from without. Retention of a natural evacuation or resorption of matter prepared for excretion, only represents defective sewerage occurring within the body; and possibly, in a low condition of vitality producing those same injurious influences from which fever is known to be developed, wherever a feeble frame is exposed to the noxious emanations arising from decomposing animal matter.

Vicarious Menstruation.—As menstruation consists in an effectual fulfilment of the series of special functional changes

---

[1] Essay on the Chlorosis of Boarding Schools.

already described, it is evident that the substitution of a channel of relief, vicarious to the process of uterine evacuation, must be considered as a form of amenorrhœa. Practically, there is a wide difference between these cases and those in which the energies of the body are elsewise employed; as in convalescence from exhaustive disease — where the determining influence (always antecedent to any local impulse) has ceased to operate. In vicarious menstruation the process makes a certain progress at each period; the patient generally recognises the occurrence of those symptoms which denote approach of the menstrual epoch, and even learns to take these as a warning of the threatening vicarious relief. There is no arrest in the order of constitutional change and natural ovulation; but there is partial or entire check of the uterine efflux. The agencies which determine the filling of the vessels of the womb act with full force, and it would be only in accordance with the history of other mechanical hæmorrhages, due to hepatic or cardiac obstruction, if effusion of blood occurred at the antecedent part which presented least resistance. The analogy is so far borne out that, in the majority of cases, vicarious menstrual hæmorrhages issue from parts immediately influenced by the portal circulation; and its very intimate relations with the uterine vessels have been already described. In cases of vicarious menstruation, the blood is most commonly passed by stool or vomited from the stomach. Where hæmatemesis happens, the patient becomes reasonably alarmed. Hence its occurrence as a vicarious method of relief, is professionally observed and recorded. But cases in which there is a passage of blood by stool—either supplementary or vicarious—are, I have reason to believe, of much more frequent occurrence than is generally supposed. The suffering which women subject to hæmorrhoids experience at their menstrual periods, marks the general tendency to portal congestion. But I have frequently noted in amenorrhœa the regular occurrence at each menstrual period of a decided attack of diarrhœa; marked by fluid stools, often by tenesmus and a sense of weight in the lower gut, but without any symptoms of intestinal irritation. In such cases patients rarely observe the character of the evacuations, or only notice that they are very loose and very dark. And as iron is somewhat indiscriminately administered, the colour is referred to its action.

In two cases of this kind, where no medicine had been administered, the patients came to me stating that they suffered from bleeding internal piles; this explanation having been afforded when they were alarmed at the appearance of blood in the motions. As in hæmorrhoids occurring in women there is always some increase of the venous congestion at the menstrual times, it is easy to understand how the rough ideas which women acquire from talking to one another about their ailments, should afford this ready explanation, though the hæmorrhage be in reality vicarious. In the cases alluded to, there was no evidence of any disease of the rectum; and the symptoms disappeared on re-establishment of the natural menstrual profluvium. The communications which exist between the uterine plexus and the general venous system have been held to sufficiently explain the discomfort endured at the menstrual period by women of full habit who suffer from varicose veins of the legs, or from the ordinary ulcers which are dependent on this unhealthy condition. These sores or " bad-legs," when occurring in women, present a marked retardation of the healing process during the term of menstruation; occasionally there is considerable vicarious hæmorrhage from the raw surface of the ulcer; or an apparently healthy cicatrix may give way even months after its healing, on any partial or entire check of menstruation. The class of patients where these conditions are most frequent, comprises principally those who " are on their feet all day long," and are exposed to extreme vicissitudes of temperature; as is the case with cooks, or in a less degree, among shop-women. This mechanical influence affords a remarkable contrast with the results which generally obtain where the occupation is altogether sedentary.

Vicarious menstruation may, in the majority of instances, be explained and successfully treated, by such prior recognition of the inter-relations of the venous circulation. But there occasionally occur cases where other and very diverse causes have to be taken into consideration. The periodicity of the hæmorrhagic flux is maintained; but it may issue from the lungs, the throat, the ears, the gums, the bladder, the nipples, the surface of the skin, or the cicatrix of an old wound. And these cases tend to strengthen the belief that every retained excretion is, *pro tanto*, a means of blood empoisonment. The local determination and efflux would, in such cases, depend upon some pre-existing organic defect. That part which is weakest soonest gives way. Vicarious menstrual hæmorrhage, whencesoever it may occur, is of very different significance from effusion of blood, the result of local disease, but it serves to direct attention to the condition of the part from which it flows, and indicates what other considerations must be borne in mind whilst it is sought to re-establish the natural order of menstruation.

MENORRHAGIA.—The restricted sense in which the term menorrhagia is now employed has followed increased attention in the diagnosis of those local organic changes which commonly induce true uterine hæmorrhage (metrorrhagia). Amenorrhœa usually occurs at an early part of the menstrual life, and most frequently is of systemic or ovarian origin. Menorrhagia is generally met with in women past the middle term of sexual life (which occurs about 32), and usually depends upon some disordered condition, either vascular, textural, or physical, of the uterus itself. The excessive flux which characterizes menorrhagia naturally attracts special attention to the uterus, whence the blood proceeds. But it is by no means rare to meet with cases where the organ itself is absolutely free from disease, yet there occurs at each month so profuse a flow as sometimes to immediately endanger life. In the whole range of the numerous disorders affecting the generative cycle, none require more vigilant care than in tracing out of the history of cases of recurring menorrhagia. Nor is the obvious immediate danger from excessive flow the only source of apprehension. Such repeated draining away of an inordinate amount of blood is most detrimental to physical vigour. The damage may not be immediately obvious, or the patient appear to soon regain her original health. But the influence is exercised on the other end of her life. The woman who repeatedly suffers from severe menorrhagia, and who permits the disorder to proceed unchecked, will become prematurely old; will, at a comparatively early period, present evidence of approaching decrepitude and of that rearrangement of nutrition already mentioned as ushering in old age.—p. 110.

The terms active and passive menorrhagia are now comparatively little employed. Practically they have no further value than as serving to steady the process of investigation by which it is sought to arrive at the true cause of the excessive flux. Periodic occurrences of menorrhagia, with an entire absence of sanguineous discharge during the intervals, and a wide variation (sometimes even an alternation) in the amount lost at successive menstrual periods, usually indicates that the efflux is due to exalted functional action, unaccompanied by organic disease. Yet it must be borne in mind that the first evidence of that tendency to uterine hæmorrhage which commonly accompanies certain structural disorders is often afforded by simple exaggeration of the menstrual flow; which thenceforth gradually increases in amount and duration. Menorrhagia is necessarily a comparative term; that which would be a natural relief to one woman constitutes an exhaustive flow in another; and a similar variation may occur at different periods of the same life. Hence it is necessary to take into account the physical condition of each patient and the circumstances of her life, and even to question somewhat closely as to the extent of the flux; for sometimes a weakly, fragile woman, suffering from functional menorrhagia will confidently state her menstruation to be natural, judging herself by the standard of some more robust friend with whom she has compared notes.

In some cases there is the history of attacks of exhaustive menorrhagia occurring at one or several periods, long intervals elapsing during which the catameniæ occur naturally; but in most cases of menorrhagia patients refrain from seeking medical assistance until alarmed by the long continuance of the excessive flux. I have notes also of several cases where the menorrhagia habitually ensued during one or two periods at certain seasons, especially in the spring or fall of the year; times when it used to be considered salutary to let blood. This ancient practice was directed for the relief of some supposed undue stress on the vascular system; and practically it is advisable in persons of plethoric habit to obviate the influence of the rapid variations of temperature at these seasons by the use of occasional saline aperients. In this way the menorrhagia was averted for two years in one of the cases above referred to, where the lady had come to consider its recurrence in the spring and autumn as constitutional and not to be safely interfered with.

The order which the excessive flux assumes in different

cases is of practical importance. In some it comes on almost suddenly, and ceases as quickly. The patient being unwilling to bestir herself through dread of the gush of blood that follows the least effort or excitement. In other cases, the menstruation follows its natural course for two or three days, and then there is a sudden and great increase without assignable cause. Sometimes the flux intermits; and I have known this effect to assume the quotidian or tertian types where a foregone ague had left no other recognisable evidence of its abiding influence. In one of these cases the original fever had been contracted in Egypt six years previously, but the patient was approaching the climacteric period. In a third group of cases the menstrual flow gradually increases day by day, from its first appearance until the exhaustion of the patient induces frequent fainting, and the pulse is scarcely perceptible. Again, there may be a natural but free flow presenting all the menstrual characters, but there ensues from time to time an expulsive effort accompanied by the passage of clots which gradually increase in size. These variations in the character of the menorrhagic flow need to be carefully considered in each case. In many the patients have gone on hoping against hope, until the excess of menstruation has so encroached on the natural intervals that the system scarcely rallies from the exhaustive effect of one period before another sets in. Here there is little time to be lost; for the risk is evident and the danger often imminent, and every point in the history is worthy of note, since the causes of menorrhagia are many and complicated.

When considering the changes which precede, determine, and accompany the occurrence of healthy menstruation, the special agency of the systemic ovarian and uterine influences were referred to in definite order. But the practical advantage of this distinction is only recognisable when it comes to be applied to the consideration of disorders of the menstrual function. As in amenorrhœa, so also in menorrhagia and dysmenorrhœa, the division adopted helps to steady the diagnosis and guide the treatment.

The Systemic Causes of Menorrhagia.—There are certain disordered conditions of the general health, or of parts holding no immediate relation with the organs constituting the female generative cycle, which tend to produce menorrhagia. Bright's disease, scurvy, purpura, and saturation with certain mineral poisons, act by vitiation of the general condition of the blood. Whatever retards or impedes the equable working off of the venous blood—such as pressure on the ascending cava, pneumonia, emphysema, tubercular deposition in the lungs, or any obstructive disease of the heart or liver—may indirectly produce menorrhagia. Rapid passage to a tropical climate often induces its occurrence; and it is advisable in cases where there is any tendency to inordinate menstruation that the long sea voyage be recommended instead of the overland route—for patients going to India or China. Many cases of menorrhagia attributed to the fatigues of the voyage are in reality due to the quick transition from a temperate to a tropical climate. So also the general excitement and unaccustomed exertion of the "wedding tour" has often more to do with the occurrence of menorrhagia early in married life than the local causes to which the untoward result is usually attributed. Women thus susceptible have frequently shown other signs of tendency to bleeding attributed to the existence of an hæmorrhagic diathesis. Menorrhagia sometimes ensues in this country from the same systemic condition. But where attributable to this cause, there is usually some notable excitability both of brain and heart. This condition must not be confounded with the excessive menstrual relief which often occurs in women of full habit who live freely and take little exercise; who feed their bodies and starve their intellects. Excessive menstruation, even to a dangerous extent, may ensue from strong mental impressions; the relation of cause and effect being just as clear as in those cases of menstrual suppression already described as dependent on mental shock. In the latter case the influence exercised is depressant; where menorrhagia ensues it is usually found that the cause has been of an excitant kind, such as vehement endeavour to accomplish something beyond the capacity, fits o. anger or passion, or long anxiety. I have in numerous instances known menorrhagia ensue in delicate women who have overtaxed both their physical and mental endurance by continuous attendance on the sick, and especially by nightwatching. Again, there are certain influences which, though physically affecting the whole system, only manifest their effects by recurring menorrhagiæ. Where the gouty diathesis is strongly marked, menstruation is usually free and sometimes excessive. The injudicious use of very hot baths, stimulants taken in excess, violent and unaccustomed exercise, and habitually living in very hot and dry rooms, may be included in this class of causes.

Menorrhagia dependent on ovarian irritation is usually associated with dysmenorrhœa of a special kind, to be hereafter described. In healthy menstruation, the uterine efflux is in response to an influence of ovarian origin. In congenital absence of the ovaries, or after their extirpation, no indication of menstrual effort ensues. Admitting this dominance of the ovarian impulse in determining menstruation, it would follow that inordinate ovarian action might exalt in a corresponding degree the uterine flow. The occasional occurrence of multiple births is only explicable on the assumption that there has been an exceptional maturation of several ova at one menstrual period; and in cases of death occurring during menstruation, examination of the ovaries has shown that there exists very considerable variation in the number of Graafian vesicles which present at different periods. After careful inquiry in a large number of cases, I am led to believe that there are very few women of middle age who have not at times noticed considerable differences in the amount and duration of the menstrual flow not referable to any recognised influences. If (other things being equal) the greater or less extent of ovulation induces a corresponding uterine determination, it is obvious that wide variations in the amount of the menstrual flow might so be produced; hence, cases of menorrhagia due to excessive sexual indulgence, in which there is usually considerable ovarian tenderness, receive a ready explanation. Just as a smooth, unwrinkled condition of the ovaries readily accounts for amenorrhœa, so the evidence of recent coincident maturation of a large number of ova might sometimes afford the explanation of those obscure cases of death from profuse menorrhagia occurring in the virgin as well as in the multiparous woman, where no evidence of real disease can be traced. In menorrhagia of ovarian origin there is always a marked tenderness on deep pressure with the finger-tips in one or both of the ovarian regions. The ovary can be recognised as larger than natural, it rolls beneath the pressure of the finger, but the change of place is accompanied with pain of a sickening character; and there is present, to an inordinate degree, that wearying dull pain in the loins which women commonly describe as a "back-ache." In the intervals (should there be a reason for instituting digital examination), the ovary on the tender side will be often distinguished as inordinately large. In some cases this condition is so marked that the uterine sound must be introduced to assure that the tumid projection which is felt by the finger does not depend on some fibro-cystic outgrowth from the womb, or on latero-flexion of the organ.

Uterine Menorrhagia, where the excessive flux arises from some disordered or diseased condition of the womb itself, comprises the majority of the cases ordinarily met with. The same result may ensue under very various conditions. It accompanies hyperplasia, as in the growth of polypi or fibrous tumours; aplasia, where the structure is destroyed by erosions or ulcerations; and cacoplasia, where the tissue-changes are of the new type presented in malignant disease. But in such cases simple periodic menorrhagia is usually a transition state, which gradually merges into a recurring hæmorrhage until all count of the menstrual period is lost. There are, in addition, certain disordered conditions of the uterine textures which acknowledge very various causes, but frequently only attract attention when repeated attacks of menorrhagia, quite periodic though very profuse, alarm the patient by their exhaustive extent. This form of uterine menorrhagia is commonly met with in women of feeble habit towards the approach of the change of life, and often follows miscarriage, or a tedious labour where the process of involution has been inefficiently performed, and an effort is made to suckle the child. It is very generally believed by women that, after a *fausse couche*, or a confinement without subsequent lactation, all will be right if only the catameniæ can be induced to recur. Hence very mischievous results too frequently ensue where means are adopted for inducing the menstrual flow, in other words, to excite to effort the imperfectly rehabilitated uterus; the usual result being an exhaustive menorrhagia of the kind now under consideration.

The patient presents those general symptoms which indicate deficiency of vital energy, of reparative force, and of physical tonicity. She is languid and feeble, tired from the least exertion, and takes long to recover from the exhaustion produced by effort; her legs swell on walking; and she complains of a dragging or sense of existent weight in the body—sometimes amounting to that which women commonly describe as a bearing down; symptoms exaggerated by standing, and often remaining for hours after any strain, as in defecation. The uterus is found, on examination, to be low down in the pelvis, heavy, soft, and of inordinate length; this being due to enlargement of the body of the organ, which is frequently found displaced. The cervix is large, the os usually patulous and easily admitting the finger. But there is no special tenderness; indeed, a steady pressure upwards, by relieving the strain on the connective supporting structures, often affords temporary relief. Such a condition is comparatively rare in the virgin, but may ensue after long continued leucorrhœa in women of relaxed habit of body. It is in cases of true passive menorrhagia that leucorrhœa chiefly occurs between the periods of excessive menstruation; and this should afford additional reason for close investigation of the history. Both are attributable to some general influence locally determined by some special cause. It is utterly erroneous to consider the leucorrhœa as " evidently the cause of the menorrhagia," or *vice versâ*.

This form of menorrhagia is far more commonly met with in large towns, and especially among the poor. From my own observation, I incline to believe that defect of uterine involution is a very frequent cause, either directly or indirectly, of a form of obstinate passive menorrhagia, readily checked by treatment, but very likely to recur with just the same severity when the next period comes round.

In these cases, the excessive flux is certainly of uterine origin, and local treatment will afford some temporary relief. Re-position of the organ, if displaced, the application of leeches, the use of potent local astringents, or even the introduction of medicated pessaries, may benefit for a while. But here the condition of the uterus is really only one of many evidences of a general diminution of structural power; and local applications, if used at all, should be merely ancillary.

In the treatment of menorrhagia, the distinction of its cause is of especial importance for the framing of a method of cure; and those inter-relations alluded to in the foregoing descriptions demand especial consideration. Where the efflux is of systemic origin, and but a passive issue of blood, it is eminently important that the drain be checked as soon as this can safely be effected. For it denotes a disarrangement of the vascular relations common to the whole body; so that other parts starve for want of that nutritive material oozing away in the blood which flows from the womb.

There are certain drugs which exercise an undoubted influence in checking such effusions, and certain combinations of them whereby their action is so steadied and guarded as to insure that the special benefit is not gained at the cost of some injurious effect elsewhere produced.

The remedies chiefly in use and most worthy of trust for the treatment of systemic menorrhagiæ, comprise the mineral acids, especially the nitric and sulphuric : certain metallic salts, of alum, iron, lead, zinc, copper, and silver; the various vegetable products which contain tannin ; or possess distinct astringent properties, as the gum-resins, matico, &c. These are commonly exhibited in full doses whilst yet the excessive flow is going on, to arrest the hæmorrhage as soon as may be, in addition to their use in the intervals. Hence it becomes important to guard their action and watch their effect, so that there may not be produced other and sometimes equally serious evils. The combination of a saline aperient, of a diaphoretic or of a diuretic, will obviate many of these; but it is always important to select that form of astringent which the general condition of the patient and state of the pulse, &c., indicates as specially suitable. Thus, in obese women, with flabby muscles and little energy, physical or mental, the vegetable astringents are especially useful after the removal of any intestinal obstruction. Matico (in the form of an alcoholic extract) is one of the most serviceable in such cases. In thin, worn women suffering from menorrhagia, the mineral acids and astringent salts are indicated. If there be great nervous irritability, full doses of sulphate of zinc (from five to eight grains) exercise a powerful influence in controlling the hæmorrhage. Where, on the other hand, the pulse is inordinately quick, and rapidly fluctuates, the acetate of lead with opium proves eminently useful. In every case the menorrhagia results from a combination of adverse conditions, and it is only from the study of these that the appropriate remedy can be selected.

Certain other drugs have from time to time been strongly recommended as of special value in the treatment of systemic menorrhagia, for example, digitalis and the oxide of silver. But statements as to the special efficacy of new remedies for menorrhagia require to be received with the utmost caution. They are usually only tried after other and ordinary means have been for some time employed without advantage, and when, therefore, the period of excessive flux is near its natural termination; so that the relief may be *post* and not *propter*. Of the drugs above mentioned both have been recommended on high authority, whilst other observers have reported their utter failure. They serve to illustrate the importance of always avoiding, in cases where life is endangered, the use of remedies about which the evidence is so widely contradictory as in the instances cited; for the oxide of silver is chemically unstable, and digitalis is therapeutically uncertain, when given medicinally.

Menorrhagia attributable to ovarian origin is so commonly preceded or accompanied by symptoms of dysmenorrhœa, that these generally first attract attention, and the excessive flux, sometimes remitting, sometimes continuous, is rightly regarded as a result of the same cause that induces the special suffering at each menstrual time. But there is a form of ovarian menorrhagia, accompanied by a sense of fulness rather than of actual pain in the ovarian regions, which I have met with as of especial occurrence in women of full habit, who have always menstruated regularly, but recognise, when past the middle age of uterine life, an increasing sense of effort at each of the periods. It is in cases of ovarian origin, in so far as the recorded histories serve as a guide, that Indian hemp principally exercises the beneficial influence attributed to it as a remedy for menorrhagia. But ovarian menorrhagia is so intimately connected with dysmenorrhœa of the same origin that the treatment will be considered under that heading.

Menorrhagia of true uterine origin rarely occurs early in life; it is most common in those who have borne children or suffered miscarriages. It so persists, and with such serious effects, that there is seldom any difficulty in ascertaining its cause. This is a class of case in which local examination is absolutely imperative. Here, as whenever the uterus has to be examined, it is important to consider the personal peculiarities of each patient. Many, even when past middle age, are so absolutely ignorant about themselves that some tact is required when it becomes necessary to explain what is wrong. Women are naturally averse to vaginal examination whilst menorrhagia is going on. If, however, there be reason to consider the hæmorrhage as strictly of uterine origin, it is the plain duty of the practitioner to thoroughly investigate the local conditions, and continue his research until the mode of the flux is made out. Where menorrhagia is due to disorder of structure, as in cases of polypus, of fibrous tumours, of caruncular or other growths, of malignant disease, the employment of local styptics, the application of cold, &c., or, in very severe cases, resort to plugging the vagina, continuous pressure on the abdominal aorta, &c., are only expedients prefatory to the particular treatment appropriate for each case so soon as the hæmorrhagic attack has been checked. (Vide ch. iv.) It has been recommended that the uterine orifice should be plugged in place of applying the sponges, as is usually done, in the upper part of the vagina. The danger of such innovation is, that dilatation of the cervix, as proved by Dr. Barnes, tends to induce expulsive effort—hence blood collected in the uterine cavity might find a vent through the Fallopian tubes, and induce peritonitis, as pointed out in the memoir of M. Bernutz.

In the cases already described, where the uterus is found large and spongy, but without any appreciable lesion of structure, local examination either directs attention to, or decides the diagnosis of, a general defect in tonicity. In some instances, especially where the patient is somewhat advanced in life, and has borne many children, the symptoms closely resemble those of the early stage of malignant disease, the cervix uteri being chronically indurated and irregular. In these cases, and where the patient is seen early, the endeavour should be so to control the flux as to bring it within the ordinary limits of natural menstruation. Rest on a hard couch, in a quiet, cool room, with the pelvis raised above the level of the shoulders and lightly covered; the application of wet cloths to the body;

the use of a nearly cold saline enema, with the administration of suitable astringents (especially the combination of tannic and sulphuric acid with opium and Epsom salts), will, in the majority of cases, suffice to effect this. Astringent vaginal injections are to be avoided at the outset, since the engorged womb might suffer from the sudden check. Alum, lead, or gallic acid are the most serviceable, and the solution should be injected in a continuous stream.[1] Where only temporary alleviation follows, the menorrhagia recurring on the least exertion or excitement, the ergot of rye often checks the drain of blood, by inducing contraction of the enfeebled uterine tissue, thus naturally closing the orifices whence the oozing occurs. Here also firm pressure, just as it is used in post-partum hæmorrhage, assists by its mechanical action. When the menorrhagia still goes on, resort must be had to more powerful local means for its arrest. Here the employment of intra-uterine injections are indicated. The judicious precaution of always assuring that the canal of the cervix is patulous before employing this method of treatment is in these cases anticipated by the relaxed structural condition of the parts; for the finger readily enters the cervical passage. I have repeatedly introduced strong solutions of perchloride of iron as a local styptic in these severe cases with no other result than that of checking profuse passive menorrhagia. The most convenient instrument

---

[1] An excellent instrument for this purpose is that French apparatus known as the "Irrigateur." It is self-acting, and the force of the stream can be very easily regulated.

is a glass syringe, having attached to it a silver tube with perforations at its bulbous end,[1] which is passed within the cervix to the depth of an inch and a half.

When the immediate flux is arrested, the setting in order of the general health demands careful attention. Hygienic treatment is especially important in those cases of exhausted vital energy frequently met with in women who have borne children very rapidly, who have resided long in hot climates, or have allowed a gradually-increasing menorrhagia to go on, sometimes for years, until the strength is broken by the long-continued drain. The employment of the cold douche each night, and of a hip-bath in the morning, provided a due reaction follow constitutes the local treatment. Dr. Gooch strongly recommended enemata of cold water, as the vaginal injection sometimes tends to induce accumulation in the rectum, by extension of its influence to the adjacent bowel. A combination of salines with the mineral tonics suffices to obviate this trouble. The value of the preparations of iron in these cases is beyond question, administered during the intervals between the attacks, and large doses can often be borne with impunity. In all cases of menstrual disorder requiring the use of this drug I have, for several years, followed the plan of administering large doses, until some indications are presented that the extreme of tolerance has been reached; giving, frequently, a drachm of the tincture of the sesquichloride three

---

[1] Made by Coxeter, Grafton-street East.

times a day, or correspondingly large doses of other suitable preparations. Wherever menorrhagia occurs, and whatever its cause, it is necessary to carefully watch the coming round of the next period, to place the patient under the most favourable conditions with special reference to the influences, whether systemic, ovarian, or uterine, which are recognised to have been at fault on previous occasions.

The scraping of the interior of the uterus with a sharp-edged curette, for relief of obscure menorrhagia, is a haphazard process, utterly unjustifiable, being both unscientific and dangerous. It has proved of service in some cases by the vehement mechanical irritation inducing uterine contraction. But this latter result may be attained by other means, and without the serious risk incurred by blindly scraping the delicate and peculiarly organized tissue which lines the body of the uterus.

DYSMENORRHŒA.—The cases included under this title comprise all those where menstruation is attended with distinctive suffering; whether confined to the generative cycle, or so far outgoing any indications of local pain that the latter is disregarded by the patient when describing her symptoms. Difficult menstruation represents an exaggeration of the conditions of *malaise* always more or less associated with the recurrence of the "poorly times" in even healthy women. Some passing languor, or slight feverishness; irritability, or inability, either mental or physical; some tendency to nausea or other digestive derangement; some distinctive pain either of back or body, or the special recurrence at these periods of headache, tic-douloureux, or toothache; of dysuria, of hæmorrhoids or other slighter ailments, represent, each of them, a condition which, carried to its extreme, may become a distinctive source of intense suffering. To afford relief, it is of primary importance that the special association of the symptoms be regarded throughout. The majority of authors, as Mons. Dugès observes, recognise in dysmenorrhœa a term only applicable when real uterine pains occur. But the word dysmenorrhœa, if its pure and simple meaning be accepted, very fairly indicates what is necessary to be considered; and the restriction of its use to cases where the symptoms are local, would lead to the exclusion of a large and important group. Even on a more liberal interpretation of the term, it has been held sufficient to consider all cases of marked suffering at the menstrual periods as either neuralgic, congestive, or mechanical. But the cases are very exceptional where either of these conditions is entirely absent; or in which it would be judicious to conduct the treatment with exclusive regard to neuralgia, congestion, or mechanical obstruction. The adverb δὺς is an inseparable particle; it exactly expresses some untoward condition, some accompanying difficulty concurrent with the menstrual period; and, unless this association be recognised in all its bearings, the diagnosis must be confused, and the treatment unsatisfactory. The same method hitherto adopted in considering menstruation and its disorders, appears applicable for the distinction of cases of dysmenorrhœa.

Systemic Dysmenorrhœa.—The various functional processes which specially minister to the continuance of life have a close co-ordination evidently intended to insure uniformity of action; all the structures or organs which assist in the carrying out of any one process being grouped together under one common control. The ganglionic system of nerves, the Præsidium of Nutrition, appears to be principally charged with this work of adjustment, and the distribution of its stations of communication, or ganglia, favours this view. Those processes which involve rapid and constant nutritive changes, or where absolute precision of action is essential to due fulfilment of function, are thus especially guided and governed; the nerve distribution corresponding to the vital importance of each. Digestion, circulation, aëration, elimination, reproduction, and the special senses, especially illustrate such endowments. The several ganglionic centres are in direct communication with sensory nerves, but under healthy conditions these convey no sense of the constant changes they control further than those test-conditions of normal communication, well illustrated by the recurring feeling of hunger and sense of satiety. There may occur an exaggeration of this sensory apprehension, so that, without any actual disorder in the special organ, or groups of organs, to which the feeling is referred, the natural changes unfelt in health are recognised as sources of *malaise* or suffering. Hypochondriasis and hysteria are probably attributable to such a condition. The differences presented in the personal appreciation of slight functional disorders, and the general susceptibility to pain, vary widely in different persons, and at different times in the same individual; hence the importance of ascertaining, as nearly as may be, whether absolute and indubitable suffering, such as occurs in cases of dysmenorrhœa, really arises from some local disorder or is due to morbid general hyperæsthesia.

The female generative cycle either generally or in any one of its parts may thus induce a series of subjective symptoms having a very wide range; whilst the local processes are fulfilled in exact order. In such cases it is important to carefully discriminate the relation of the local changes and the general symptoms, and especially to guard against the belief that because suffering occurs at the menstrual periods, therefore the organs then specially in active operation are necessarily at fault. In women of an exceptionally excitable nature, or in whom there have at times occurred indications of mental derangement, the period of menstruation is often accompanied by evidences of inordinate cerebral excitement, requiring very assiduous care. There may be only such excessive sensitiveness that the patient cannot bear light or sound or mental effort, and at each period shuts herself out as far as possible from external impressions; or the term may be accompanied by so extreme an exaggeration of these symptoms that the reason is suborned, and there accrues a condition which is, for the time, little different from mental aberration. Where symptoms thus marked occur early in life, and especially if there be any hereditary tendency to insanity, marriage should be positively prohibited. It may be that a careful investigation of the physical relations will enable a cure to be effected; but it is well ascertained that those who become pregnant whilst the functional nervous relations are thus periodically disturbed are peculiarly liable to suffer from puerperal mania in its most severe form.

It is a point worthy of note, that in these conditions of extreme mental excitement concurrent with the menstrual period, women are usually less susceptible to the physical influences which, under ordinary circumstances, would probably produce immediate suppression and its attendant ills. In one case which came under my care, the patient, a single lady, had on two occasions walked barefoot in the gardens at night in winter, gesticulating wildly. She returned to the house at the solicitations of her maid, slept long and soundly, and when she woke the menstruation was still going on naturally.

Cases of this kind represent an influence clearly associated with the local changes. Confirmation of this intense sympathy may also be found in the records of those numerous authenticated instances where women during the period of pregnancy have presented a changed nature, have been guilty of revolting crimes, or exhibited indubitable signs of temporary insanity. These influences should be borne in mind in all cases of female insanity occurring during active uterine life; in fact, no woman should be accredited as insane until the influences above described have been carefully investigated and any exaggerating local disorder removed.

In cases of epilepsy in women, the frequency with which

the seizures occur at menstrual periods (usually preceding "the show") has not received the attention it deserves. The inquiries appear to have been chiefly directed to ascertain coincidence of local uterine disorder; and there is considerable variance in the results given by careful observers. Dr. Reynolds says, " The complications of epilepsy which exist in the uterine system are of no very definite character, and they lead to no practical conclusion with regard to the convulsive affection."[1] Dr. Aitken states that, " Irregularity and perverted state of the menstrual function, associated with hysteria, is a frequent source of the malady."[2] In three cases of epilepsy under my notice, the fits, which had recurred for several years, always ensued at the time of menstruation, there being no local dysmenorrhœal symptoms at these menstrual periods when no seizures occurred. In numerous other instances the attacks ensued at or immediately prior to the menstrual periods more frequently than at any other time. In one of these cases there was amenorrhœa of two years' continuance, caused by accidental exposure and cold; but the epileptic attacks recurred with singular regularity about the times when the menstruation would have been due. The re-establishment of the natural flow was accompanied by a fit of unusual intensity. In very many other cases the seizures notably occurred at, or just previous to, the menstrual periods; but the frequency with which the patients suffered from similar fits during the

---

[1] Epilepsy, p. 236.   [2] Science of Medicine, vol. ii. p. 536.

intervals excludes these cases from consideration, except as affording corroborative testimony. The coincidence of epileptic seizures with periods of notable uterine changes, as at the time of puberty, in puerperal eclampsia, and at the change of life, corroborates the view above expressed.[1] The association between the uterine changes and spasmodic hysterical attacks should be borne in mind; for I have known immediate suppression induced by roughly pouring cold water on a girl in whom the symptoms resembled, but were correctly distinguished from, true epilepsy. Where hysteria presents this convulsive aspect in women, the attacks generally occur at the catamenial period. With the improved system of training now so generally adopted with girls, we may expect that hysterical simulation and other cases where reason and judgment are suborned, and morbid impressions allowed to acquire an exaggerated and mischievous influence, will continue to diminish in number. That true hysteria, which acquired its name from the systemic influence of the uterine changes, will necessarily occur, but most other forms of this malady are traceable to some disregard of ordinary hygienic conditions. Distinct from hysteria is a form of suffering occasionally met with at the menstrual times, where the processes are effected naturally and healthily, but where the great periodic distress often leads to the suspicion that there must be some existing local disease. These

---

[1] " Solet denique hæc passio pubertatis tempore, sive novæ purgationis in fæminis aut prime partus quadam naturali."—*Cælius Aurelianus.* (u.c. 200).

patients are neither hysterical nor in the ordinary sense nervous, are not feeble of body, and are usually endowed with mental powers above the average. But they are especially impressionable; recognise little differences which others do not observe; enjoy more intensely all pleasurable things, whether appealing to the intellectual or sensory faculties; but suffer also, both in mind and body, to an equal degree; feel pain more acutely, and feel as pain what produces in others a scarcely recognisable discomfort.

The conditions hitherto described include a considerable portion of the cases commonly referred to neuralgic dysmenorrhœa. It must, however, be borne in mind that neuralgia really means nothing; a patient complains of nervous pain; telling her that it is neuralgia is only translating her words into Greek. Where the susceptibility to influences originating in the generative cycle is of less extent there accrue a variety of symptoms which may be conveniently considered as purely sympathetic; neither exaggerated nor controlled by any exercise of the mental faculties. It may be that the coming on of menstruation is marked by extreme sensitiveness in other ganglionic centres; that there is, at such times only, pain after food, urgent vomiting, hepatic derangement, the deep lumbar-ache of renal irritation, "uterine asthma," or unwonted sense of the heart's action without any appreciable derangement of the organs to which the symptoms are specially referred. Beyond these, and indicating an influence exercised on the sensory nerves, are the severe headaches which so commonly attend difficult menstruation. They accord very precisely with those which arise when any of the co-ordinate processes already mentioned are disturbed in their working, or where their changes are appreciated with undue sensitiveness. The intense brow-ache, the sense of tenderness referred to one or other side of the head; the sharp darting pains which remit but do not cease, and especially occur in the temples between the eyes and at the vertex, ensue or are exaggerated in severity at the menstrual periods. The common periodic sick-headache to which women are especially liable, in many cases invariably precedes the occurrence of the catamenia. In one such case, of fifteen years' duration, the patient was only free from her habitual headaches during the times of pregnancy.

In all the cases above referred to the influence becomes proportionally exaggerated if any local derangement ensue, or the existing susceptibility be intensified by the presence of actual uterine disease, or by injudicious local treatment. The effect of injuries, intestinal obstruction, tight lacing, urgent vomiting, or other violent efforts at the menstrual period, may interrupt or interfere with the process, and produce dysmenorrhœal suffering, sometimes of very intense kind. It sometimes happens that the symptoms are very persistently referred to the uterine region, though no local disorder exists; here great caution is requisite. For it cannot be denied that there occasionally come under notice unhappy cases where an ill-regulated mind, a morbid susceptibility, an injudicious or even vicious training, has induced unrestrained indulgence in sensual or erotic ideas, even without any direct physical impurity. The discrimination of these painful cases, and the distribution of the counsel which has to be given to the patient and her friends, requires much tact and grave consideration. It may be a professional duty to warn and guide; but it would be an obvious breach of a very delicate trust if by any ambiguous expression, unguarded phrase, or suggestive cross-questioning the patient were led to concentrate her attention on sensations already productive of morbid influence.

The treatment of the wide range of cases above described under the head of systemic dysmenorrhœa obviously demands that attention should be directed to the general rather than to the local symptoms. The employment of suitable sedatives and other means, hygienic and medicinal, may suffice to relieve the temporary suffering; but the measure of success can only be learnt when the next period comes round. By holding out this hope of alleviation, patients may often be induced to attend perseveringly to the treatment enjoined during the intervals; for it is too commonly believed that, in order to escape the habitual suffering, it is only necessary to seek advice just previous to or during menstruation.

Ovarian Dysmenorrhœa.—The occurrence of extreme tenderness in either ovarian region, and of severe dysmenorrhœal suffering referred to that spot where the pain is felt, by no means includes all the cases where difficulty in menstruation is due to irregular, disordered, or obstructed ovulation. In his valuable work on Female Diseases, Dr. Rigby carefully distinguished this form of dysmenorrhœa, remarking that the pain is confined chiefly to a spot about an inch above the middle of Poupart's ligament, frequently extending to the back, and also down the thigh. It is of a dull and peculiarly sickening character, increased or brought on by exercise, by passage of hard fæces, and by external pressure on examination. On making internal examination, either by vagina or rectum, there is intense suffering when the tender ovary is touched, and generally a definite rounded tumour is felt, as though this sensitive ovary were swollen.

True ovarian dysmenorrhœa appears to be naturally divisible into three kinds. This distinction is so far useful that it may serve to direct attention to the character of the preponderating symptoms in each case, and give precision to the method of treatment. The Neuralgic, Capsular, and Stromal forms of ovarian dysmenorrhœa are each distinguished by special symptoms; but it is rare to meet with either of these varieties existing alone and uncomplicated.

1. *True ovarian neuralgia* may continue to recur during many successive menstrual periods without any notable influence being produced either on the character, the progress, or the duration of the discharge. It sometimes ensues during the intervals, and may come to be such a source of suffering that any excitement, unwonted exertion, or deviation from the usual method of life leads to an attack, supplementary to that which always ushers in the menstrual change. The remittent pain has that special lancinating and suddenly intense character to

which it has been found convenient that the term neuralgia should be exclusively restricted, and very precisely resembles neuralgia of the testis. The patient fears to straighten the leg of the affected side, or to venture on any movement that may jar the part. The pain darts to the back, and often induces that special character of sensation so commonly described in identical terms by persons suffering from neuralgia, whatever its origin—it is an "opening and shutting pain;" and the pathological significance of this very generally used expression seems to indicate a culmination of sensory impulse, corresponding, as it has been described, to the recurring discharge of a Leyden jar. On examination, there is no notable heat or swelling, other than ordinarily accompanies the menstrual period; but the local tenderness and the local pain are often described by the patient as corresponding very precisely to that experienced in tic douloureux.

This form of dysmenorrhœa may sometimes be distinctly traced to residence in a moist climate or marshy district, and is most frequently met with in autumn. In one case it had recurred for several years at the spring and fall, with one single exception; but on this occasion, the patient (unmarried) had undergone great exertion and anxiety in nursing an invalid.

II. *In the capsular form of ovarian dysmenorrhœa*, the pain is dull, aching, and continuous, with occasional exacerbations, especially after action of the bowels, or any strain or effort. It is the character of dysmenorrhœal suffering so commonly present where there is any well-marked constitutional tendency to gout or rheumatism, and is essentially due to some special implication of the fibrous sheath which forms the capsule of the ovary. This has to be penetrated by the matured ovum; any thickening of its substances induces resistance, with a corresponding effort to overcome the obstruction, so that there may be effected that extrusion of the vesicle which represents the completed ovulation.

III. Hence it follows that *ovarian dysmenorrhœa of stromal origin* (where the structure surrounding the matured ovum carries through all the changes which should accompany extrusion, but is checked by capsular resistance) commonly accompanies that described as the second form. Here the pain is of that sickening, continuous character which can only be referred to a powerful influence, whether functional or organic, exercised on some organ immediately governed by a central plexus of the sympathetic nerve. It may be so intense that life is extinguished, as in injuries of the solar plexus; it may induce temporary intense prostration or insensibility, as in accidents affecting the liver, the kidney, or the testicle; or the impression produced may be so graduated that there ensues only the character of suffering now under consideration, as due to some undue stress on those special conditions which have for their purpose the maturation and extrusion of the ovum.

The treatment of ovarian dysmenorrhœa requires to be adjusted according to the special preponderance of one or other of the groups of symptoms above narrated, and must be regulated throughout in consideration of the attendant complications which, in practice, are found to commonly occur. In true ovarian neuralgia, the presence of hysteria has to be regarded; where the pain is referable to the capsular or fibrous element, the histories of antecedent rheumatism or gout, the state of the digestive organs, of the urine, &c., need to be specially observed. Where ovarian dysmenorrhœa is of stromal origin, there is disturbance of the special apparatus which controls the development and progress of the ova, and the irritation induces certain uterine changes which are of great importance, and will presently come to be considered.

In the first, or neuralgic form, local applications of heat and sedatives, as by the laudanum flannel, and especially by that admirable method of directing the vapour from sedative herbs adopted by Dr. Downing,[1] are eminently useful. If the pain radiate from the left ovary, a sedative injection, per rectum, will often give ease; or one of the stronger solutions of aconite, known as Liston's or Fleming's, may be painted on the affected side. As a rule, it is more expedient to adopt these local methods of treatment than to resort to sedatives administered by the mouth, whereby the whole system is influenced in order to afford relief from a pain that is purely local. Where immediate applications do not suffice to give ease, the administration of chloroform, carefully guarded and watched, will certainly allay pain, and induce sleep. The hypodermic injection of morphia, or its combination in

---

[1] Jacksonian Prize Essay on Neuralgia (1850).

a draught with chloric ether; the administration of aconite, veratria, belladonna, camphor, and stramonium, appear to exercise a beneficial influence in subduing the suffering, and allowing a period of ease or sleep during which the exaggerated sensibility becomes diminished.

These resources have, not unfrequently, to be used as supplementary to the direct treatment requisite where the ovarian dysmenorrhœa is of the second form,—of fibro-capsular origin. The common concurrence of rheumatism and neuralgia here finds additional illustration; but in such cases the diathetic symptoms especially demand attention. Large doses of the iodide or bromide of potassium, combined with the citrate of potass, have afforded very signal relief in cases where the symptoms indicated the fibrous sheath as chiefly involved; their employment, conjointly with occasional administration of colchicum, and the local application of a strong solution of iodine externally, if there be any tenderness or enlargement perceptible during the intervals, appears to furnish the most reliable method of treatment.

In the stromal variety of ovarian dysmenorrhœa it is necessary to diminish, as far as may be, the local congestion which heralds the pain, and the susceptibility which makes this delicately-organized body so sensitive after reiterated irritation. So far as the recorded histories of cases of ovarian dysmenorrhœa are intelligible, it may be judged that the existence of the neuralgic form has little or no influence on the occurrence of impregnation—that the capsular variety may occur at any period of married life, and the woman is likely thenceforth to be barren during its continuance, although she may have had children previously—that the stromal variety induces absolute sterility, which continues so long as the symptoms already described attend the menstrual periods, and until the ovarian maturation is naturally accomplished. Among those direct sedatives which appear to be especially useful, the Indian hemp occupies the first place. Combined with carbonate and hydrochlorate of ammonia in solution, it gave absolute relief in six out of eight cases where the symptoms were sufficiently clear to enable an exact diagnosis of the cause of ovarian dysmenorrhœa to be made. This affection most frequently implicates the left ovary; and it is especially important here, as in all cases of ovarian dysmenorrhœa occurring on the left side, to ascertain the ordinary character of the fæcal evacuations. It may be reported that the bowels act daily, yet a vaginal examination teaches that the rectum is charged with hard fæcal matter. The patient, having by hard straining passed a few scybalæ, is satisfied; whilst the remaining contents of the rectum continually surge and press against the tender ovary. The best aperient, in such cases, consists of a powder of sulphur, dried sulphate of magnesia, and an aromatic, stirred smoothly in a cup of warm milk, and taken each morning until the rectum no longer contains fæces.

In the intervals, when there frequently recurs a painful and sickening sensation on any effort or strain, what the patient calls "a bruised feeling," especially induced by pressure on the tender ovum, the application of two or three successive blisters to the back or groin affords great relief; combined with the internal administration of bromide of potassium and small doses of mercury, as in the pil. hydrarg. chloridi comp. Subsequently the daily use of hip-baths of real or artificial sea water proves beneficial; a loose dress, care in diet, and marital abstinence being enjoined for a time.

Uterine Dysmenorrhœa.— Cases of chronic dysmenorrhœa where the local suffering continues to periodically recur through every change of season, of climate, or mode of life, are usually of uterine origin.

There are three varieties of the disorder proper to the uterus —the Neurotic, Structural, and Obstructive; the latter including the majority of the cases described as mechanical. But there is a fourth condition where uterine pain is the chief suffering; yet the organ itself is physically and functionally healthy. Of these four forms of uterine dysmenorrhœa, two were originally described by English physicians; the first, by Dr. Gooch, the fourth by Dr. Rigby. Yet Dr. Bernutz, the latest French authority on the subject, asserts that English writers restrict local application of the term to cases which result from congenital atresia.

1. *The neurotic form* of uterine dysmenorrhœa usually attends that condition of local hyperæsthesia described by Dr. Gooch as "the irritable uterus." A patient so suffering "complains of pain in the lower part of the abdomen, along the brim of

the pelvis, and often also in the loins. The pain is worse when she is up and taking exercise, and less when she is at rest in the horizontal posture. It is always present in some degree, and paroxysms often occur although the patient has been recumbent for a long time. If the uterus is examined it is found to be exquisitely tender, the neck and body feel slightly swollen. Excepting, however, this tenderness, and occasionally this swelling, or rather tension, the uterus feels perfectly natural in structure; there is no evidence of scirrhus in the neck, the orifice is not mis-shapen, its edges are not indurated. The paroxysms generally come on either a few days before menstruation or (as is the case in many instances) a few days afterwards. The general circulation is but little disturbed; the pulse is soft, and not much quicker than is natural, but it is easily quickened on the slightest emotion. A patient who was originally delicate, who has suffered long, and has used much depleting treatment, has been " (as might reasonably be expected) " the most reduced; she has grown thin, pale, weak, and nervous; menstruation often continues regularly, but sometimes diminishes or ceases altogether. The appetite is not good, and the bowels require aperients; yet nothing more surely occasions a paroxysm of pain than an active purgative."[1]

It seems probable that certain of the cases formerly attributed to an irritable uterus were really assignable to other causes; some of ovarian origin, some due to recurring

---

[1] Gooch, Diseases peculiar to Women.

mechanical irritation, to partial displacement, or to disease of the lining membrane of the uterus. The speculum and sound are invaluable aids in assuring certainty, but should only be resorted to in cases of doubt. I fully concur in the remarks of Dr. F. W. Mackenzie, that "the clinical history of these cases, coupled with the results of treatment, give a peremptory refutation to statements on the subject which would not only identify these cases with the existence of inflammation and ulceration of the cervix uteri, but would assert the indispensable necessity of specific topical measures for their cure." Cases of irritable uterus as described by Dr. Gooch, and causing severe dysmenorrhœa where there is no structural change in any part or organ of the generative cycle, no heat, swelling, or lesion, do occasionally occur, but are probably less frequent, since greater attention has been paid to hygienic treatment. It is no longer the rule that maturing girls are laid on their backs for months to correct spinal debility, and have their chests cased in iron or whalebone until the respiration becomes perforce principally diaphragmatic: means whereby many a woman was condemned to life-long misery; an irritable uterus being only one of many forms of suffering which ensued.

Cases of true uterine dysmenorrhœa of neurotic origin may be usually traced back either to causes such as those above mentioned, to some previous exhaustive illness, or long continued anxiety, to the debility resulting from neglected leucorrhœa or from over-suckling, to ill-assorted marriage, or to irregularity of habits, either physical or social. This disorder may result from such self-sacrifice as many excellent and pure-minded women make under a sense of duty—devoting their lives to deeds of charity; but it may be equally entailed by a career of fashionable dissipation and continuous self-indulgence, pursued until "the toiling pleasure sickens into pain." For in both cases there is an over-taxing of the nervous energies.

The treatment of these cases of chronic uterine dysmenorrhœa, exclusively of nervous origin, is pretty nearly identical in principle with that advised in the first or neuralgic form of ovarian dysmenorrhœa. Here also due regard is to be paid to the occasional complication of hysteria; and the relief of the severe pains should, if possible, be effected by local means, so as to avoid the general depression which even the best-chosen sedatives, administered by mouth for relief of exclusively local pain, are likely to produce. The introduction up to the cervix uteri of a pledget of cotton wool saturated with a solution of aconitine, morphia, or extract of belladonna rubbed down with glycerine, or the use of the sedative vaginal suppositories, especially where a few drops of chloroform can be placed in the hollow of the pellet,[1] affords more decided relief than the employment of vaginal injections, since the action is more continued. The local application of chloroform vapour, recommended by Dr. Hardy,[2] is especially serviceable, since the patient can use it without trouble and without danger; or it

---

[1] These are prepared by Duncan and Flockhart, of Edinburgh.
[2] Dublin Quarterly Journal, Nov. 1853.

may be much more effectually applied by means of Dr. Downing's apparatus (p. 170), a sponge saturated with chloroform being placed in the metal chamber. In unmarried and young women, or whilst the menstrual flux is present, the same local effect may be attained by injections per rectum, with a small ball and pipe as ordinarily used (the quantity not exceeding half an ounce), or by introduction of the sedative suppositories of the Pharmacopœia. Relief is derived from the external application of hot dry flannels—sprinkled with laudanum just before contact with the abdomen—but the effect is neither so thorough nor so permanent as that obtained by the other means advised. Local depletion, as by leeching, &c., will often afford temporary relief, but the cases are not those in which loss of blood can be borne; and the present ease is attained at the cost of future suffering.

In the intervals of the periods, or as soon as the local irritability is somewhat lessened, the morning use of saline hip baths, careful regulation of the dress so as to insure mechanical rest to the uterus (p. 45), daily administration of a saline aperient, in order that no hard fæces shall press on the tender part, are means of direct influence. But the conditions which originally promoted this local suffering often necessitate a thorough investigation into the history of each case; and it is far better to wait the issue of such research than to rest content with the adoption of any pre-advised plan of treatment. I never met with two instances of irritable uterus accompanied by dysmenorrhœa identically similar in history or symptoms, and the recorded cases point to the same conclusion. The condition of the digestive organs is of special importance. The state of the tongue affords evidence as to the organs constituting the upper digestive cycle, the stomach, liver, pancreas, &c. The presence of oxalates, of lithic acid in excess, or of earthy phosphates in the urine, would indicate some error in elimination. But in every case it is desirable to ascertain all the data with as much precision as possible, and so avoid that reproach which has for centuries detracted from the dignity of medical science; for it is too commonly held that correct diagnosis only means a shrewd guess. The entire change of habits and life afforded by a residence at one or other of the ferruginous spas is of especial service in many of these cases. Careful regulation of the diet; the administration of oxide of silver, hydrocyanic acid, or bismuth, if there be gastric irritability; the use of ignatia amara or nux vomica, if there be sluggish chylopoietic action; of hydrochlorate of ammonia, podophylline and taraxacum, &c., where the liver is inactive; of nitro-muriatic acid, if there be oxalates or earthy phosphates in the urine; of scammony, if the motions be hard and dry; of aloes, if there be defective action in the large intestine. All these remedies of recognised efficacy may further require to be supplemented by agents exercising influence on the particular constitution of the individual. Quinine, iron (especially the pyrophosphate), arsenic, iodine, aconite, and zinc, are, separately or in combination, medicines having special value. But the selection must be determined by a careful following out of the history of each case; especially diverting the patient's mind from dwelling on the local ailment if there be no direct physical symptoms indicating implication of the uterus.

II. *Uterine dysmenorrhœa, of structural origin*, may accompany any one of the disordered tissue-changes hereafter to be mentioned (ch. iv.); but cases occur where structural disease, even of malignant character, attended with absence or excess of the menstrual efflux, runs its whole course unaccompanied by special dysmenorrhœal suffering. It is one of the notable things in the history of ovarian tumours, that there is rarely any account of foregone dysmenorrhœa. In the first hundred cases of ovariotomy performed by Mr. Spencer Wells, as recorded in his valuable work, there was a history of dysmenorrhœal suffering in only one instance; and here it was evidently independent of the ovarian disease.*

The suffering which frequently attends enlargement of a fibrous tumour or polypus of the uterus, is indubitably due to the mechanical interference exercised by its presence. That gradual and gentle action which, in health, insures a steady draining away of the menstrual fluid, as secerned from the lining surface, is interrupted, and pain results. The suffering which usually attends some defect of structural reparation (equally comprising simple denudation of mucous membrane and malignant ulcerative disease), may be attributed

---

* Diseases of the Ovaries, vol. i. p. 253.

in part to the periodic congestion; but in other cases, and where menorrhagic flux affords no relief, it is probably due to the expulsive uterine effort straining the sore and irritable cervix. The progressive increase of dysmenorrhœal suffering, the reference of pain to the uterine region, the local tenderness on external examination, the presence of distinctive discharges in the intervals of menstruation, and the frequent concurrence of profuse menorrhagia, justify careful examination of the state of the uterus. Where structural disorder is found to exist, the treatment must be adjusted with reference to that only, since the dysmenorrhœal pain will only cease after removal of its cause. It is to be remembered that this cessation of suffering is often gradual. I have notes of cases where uterine polypi were removed, granular sores healed, ulcerations healthily cured, yet pain still ensued for several succeeding menstrual periods, but with notable diminution as each term came round.

III. *Obstructive Uterine Dysmenorrhœa.* — The majority of cases of local dysmenorrhœal suffering, a large proportion of those where married women remain sterile,* and nearly all which are held to be of mechanical origin, depend on such an obstruction of the passage of the cervix, that the contents of the uterus are only expelled after an inordinate effort which induces pain. This narrowing may be due to some deviation of position, or it may be congenital, may follow local injury during labour, or ensue from the injudicious application

---

* In cases of sterility, Octavius Horatianus advises that it be ascertained whether the os uteri is turned aside or shut up.

of caustics to the cervix. But it may also be of true spasmodic origin; where the partial closure and consequent obstruction varies at different periods, according to the condition of the general health.

The obstruction usually occurs at either the internal or external os. I believe this is exclusively the case where obstructive dysmenorrhœa happens in women who have not borne children; but occlusion occasionally follows physical injury during labour and may be located in any part of the canal of the cervix, as will be presently described.

The pain which attends obstructive dysmenorrhœa is very precisely referred to the uterus. It is usually most intense at the commencement of the period, but may only ensue after the flow has lasted for some days. There may be but a few hours of suffering; yet sometimes it recurs for many days, until the patient is worn out with its severity, and each menstrual period is literally a time of travail. If simply due to an effort made to overcome obstruction, the vehement forcing and grinding pains sometimes recur with the regularity of those of labour, and with equal intensity, so that the patient will writhe in agony, and strain with clenched hands and set teeth as though in the throes of child-bearing. The term "uterine colic" has not inaptly been used to describe the nature of this suffering. In cases of extreme severity, where the patient appears almost convulsed by the vehemence of the pain, there is usually some accompanying ovarian complication of one or other of the forms already described.

The dysmenorrhœal suffering which commonly accompanies uterine flexion is probably in great degree attributable to the mechanical obstruction caused by the bend occurring at the junction of the body and cervix of the uterus. Occlusion of the external os, either congenital, following cicatrization of ulcers on the cervix, or caused by severe local treatment, approximates to the obstructive conditions which narrow, and sometimes render impermeable, the vaginal passage. If the closure be entire, whatever its cause and wherever its site, each recurrence of the dysmenorrhœal symptoms is accompanied by a serious danger, which has of late years received special attention. The expulsive efforts to clear away what is retained within the uterine cavity increase in vehemence as the secretion accumulates, until a passage is at last forced; and the life or death of the woman may depend upon which of the uterine orifices first gives way. Except under conditions of erethism, the uterine orifices of the Fallopian tubes are carefully guarded by sphincter tissues which contract as the uterus contracts, and therefore exercise almost a valvular influence in preventing retrogression. In pregnancy, the gradual development of muscular structure keeps up this guardianship, in addition to the resistent influence of the decidua vera. Where the uterus is gradually distended by retained menstrual fluid, no such development of its wall-tissue occurs. Under the strong contractile action which accompanies each menstrual period, the retained menses act like a fluid wedge, and the contents of the womb may be forced through one or both of the

Fallopian tubes into the cavity of the peritoneum. "This escape immediately gives rise to inflammation of the serous surface, and is characterized by some symptoms peculiar to this variety of peritonitis. There is first the time and circumstance of its occurrence; secondly, the formation immediately after of a pelvic tumour or tumours in close relation to the uterus; and thirdly, the accession of severe pain in and about the pelvis, especially in the iliac fossæ."* M. Velpeau records a case of pelvic hæmatocele which M. Bernutz adduces as evidence that " Professor Velpeau, long before the pretended discovery of hæmatocele in 1849" (by M. Nélaton), " had made out during life the diagnosis of intra-pelvic blood tumours." In the three chapters of Aëtius devoted to the consideration of pelvic abscess,† he says that " if the tumour consists of an eruption of blood, it is to be treated by applying a cautery to the most prominent spot in place of using the scalpel."

Occlusions of the cervix from injury during labour differ from congenital cases, in so far that there is an ascertained foregone full development of the organs; whereas in congenital cases the malformation of the uterus or vagina may be of such kind that any operation for establishing a passage *per vias naturales* is necessarily attended with risk. Spasmodic contraction usually occurs at the inner orifice of the canal of the cervix, and frequently accompanies ovarian dysmenorrhœa. There is a

---

* Bernutz and Goupil, Clinical Memoirs on Diseases of Women.
† Aëtius, lib. viii. ch. 85, 86, and 87.

notable variation (not present in other forms of obstructive dysmenorrhœa) as to the extent and intensity of the pain at different menstrual periods. In these cases the chief suffering is just at the commencement of menstruation; but any excitement may induce its recurrence during the period. It appears to correspond in some degree to spasmodic stricture of the urethra.

The treatment of all forms of obstructive dysmenorrhœa consists in producing and maintaining a sufficiently patulous condition of the vagina and cervical passages to allow free escape of the menstrual fluid; and it is in the latter instances, and these only, that local operative procedure in cases of sterility is justifiable. But, even then, it is right the patient should be informed why the relief accrues, that the obstruction to the menstrual efflux indicates also the cause of hindrance of impregnation. The purpose of the woman does not affect the duty of her attendant; indeed, professional respectability needs to be very carefully guarded just now, for the office of Pandarus of Troy was honourable compared with some of the procedures that have been recommended for the relief of sterility.

To remedy obstructive dysmenorrhœa, it is an essential preliminary that the nature and position of the constriction be carefully gauged. In cases of vaginal occlusion, great assistance is afforded by rectal examination, the bladder being previously emptied. It may be necessary in a congenital case to have the bladder injected by an assistant, whilst the effect is observed with the double touch, so that the precise course of the occluded vagina may be recognised. Vaginal atresia, of this extent, unless distinctly referred to some very exceptional condition which has induced the growing together of the parietes, usually accompanies deficiency of uterine development. There may be a very distinct recognition of the menstrual molimen, for the ovaries are not implicated; but the danger incurred in establishment of a vaginal thoroughfare to the uterus, and the slight chance of any subsequent result at all commensurate with the present risk, generally deters from any attempt at operation. Occlusion of the external os is readily cured when the symptoms of obstructive dysmenorrhœa can be distinctly traced to its presence. The introduction of a sponge-tent usually suffices, but where the contraction recurs after thorough dilatation, then division is the only remaining resource. The same cautious method should be pursued in all cases of organic stricture of the canal of the cervix, wherever it presents. For notwithstanding the recent strong advocacy of the use of the hysterotome, it is undoubtedly true that some amount of risk attends the operation, and that serious results have ensued even in the most skilful hands. The principle of the instrument is identical with that of the bistoire-cachée figured by Scultetus among uterine instruments (page 15). There have been numerous recent modifications, but I believe that Sir J. Y. Simpson's original hysterotome is still chiefly employed by practitioners. Messrs. Whicker and Blaise have recently constructed for me, with great skill, a metrotome, which, although not thicker

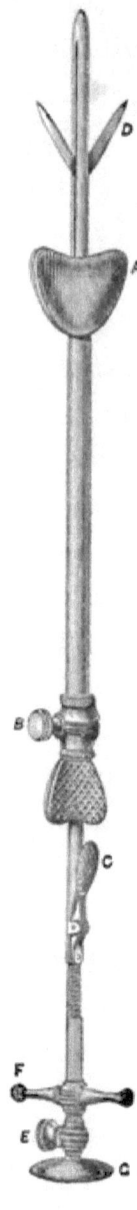

than a cedar-pencil, enables the closest stricture to be passed and bilaterally divided to any required extent without the speculum being necessary, and without extending the incision beyond the site of obstruction. The instrument is here represented. *

IV. *Membranous Dysmenorrhœa.* — Here the symptoms resemble those of obstructive dysmenorrhœa, though the structure and action of the uterus (to which the symptoms are chiefly referred) may be perfectly normal. There is formed within the uterus a fibrinous membrane, which may pass away in white shreds, or be extruded as a perfect cast of the outline of the cavity. So close is its resemblance to the decidua vera, that the name of menstrual decidua

---

* A. This guard (moving with the tube A B) is adjusted by the screw at B, to assure that the knives only open out where the stricture exists, as previously ascertained by measurement with the sound. It is to be so arranged that the guard A absolutely touches the cervix uteri when the instrument is introduced. The extent to which the knives D are to project is regulated by the nut E. The knives are brought into operation by drawing down the bar F. They cut only to a determined extent; so far as this traction is continued conjointly with that of the thumb-rest G. If division be required through the external os, then the knives sheath themselves within the guard A. If a partial stricture is to be divided, the blades may be immediately closed by pressing upwards the bar F after division of the obstruction, the catch c preventing any retrograde movement of the knives. (One-half of size of instrument.)

has been aptly applied; and it is sometimes difficult to diagnose, from mere appearances, whether the result proceeds from dysmenorrhœa, or from an early abortion. Morgagni drew attention to these exudations and to this source of error,* and Dr. Denman was so struck by the frequency of the exudations, that he believed this membrane to be produced in every case of dysmenorrhœa. " From the supposition that the membrane is always expelled, and that it consists of coagulable lymph exuded from the lining of the uterus, necessarily resulting from inflammatory action, has arisen a very faulty opinion of the nature of the disease, and a most mistaken and pernicious mode of treatment when universally applied."†

The occurrence of this form of membranous exudation was referred to its true cause by Dr. Rigby, who pointed out its coincidence with indubitable symptoms of ovarian dysmenorrhœa. I believe it most frequently accompanies that form described as stromal (p. 169). The extent and kind of action which the uterus takes on at a catamenial period is powerfully influenced by the nature of the ovarian changes. Whenever there ensues impregnation of an ovum, the subservience of the uterus is immediately evinced by the production of a lining decidual membrane, even though the germ never enters the organ, but is abnormally developed. Under conditions of ovarian irritation, or inflammation, it is conceivable how an exaggerated nerve-impression may mislead the uterus; but it is far better

---

* Epist. 48, art. 12.   † Sir C. Locock.

this should occasionally occur than that a fertilized ovum should pass away through want of the due responsive action which insures its uterine arrest and growth. The new membrane, thus systematically formed, becomes a foreign body so soon as produced, when it is only of dysmenorrhæal origin, and probably the continuance of the ovarian irritation tends to induce expulsive effort. It has to be got rid of as soon as may be; and this is effected through the natural contractile process by which foreign bodies are removed from the cavity of the uterus. If the patient be a multipara, the membrane may come away as a shreddy bag; if a virgin, it may remain until softened and disintegrated by the alkaline nature of the eliminated fluids, when it appears as bits of white membrane. This important and frequent form of membranous dysmenorrhœa, accompanied by local symptoms, referred especially to the uterus, affords, therefore, only a demonstration of the perfect working order of the organ. The treatment (except for relief of immediate pain) is to be directed to the source of the ovarian disorder. Any undue interference with the uterus itself would certainly produce one or other of those serious evils which follow whenever local treatment is unnecessarily employed.

LEUCORRHŒA.—Old writers comprised under the term "fluor albus" every vaginal discharge not absolutely sanguineous. Aëtius draws a tolerably accurate distinction; but in other works, ancient and mediæval, I have traced upwards of thirty designations, many of them very fanciful, applied to discharges included under this title. One of these is especially curious—"Fleurs blanches," used in France to describe leucorrhœa, accords precisely with a folk-word still employed in this country for designating menstruation: it is called the "Flowers." The terms were in common use two centuries ago,* and Dr. A. Farre thus refers to them: "The French term 'Fleurs' and the English 'Flowers' are now fallen into disuse; but they were employed in earlier times as designations of menstruation, for the purpose of suggesting that, after the example of trees, which do not bear unless the fruit is preceded by the blossom, so a woman does not become pregnant until she also has had her flowers."† It is, however, more than probable that "fleurs" and "flowers" only indicate a corruption of the original word "fluor," as generally used at the time when a Latin term was found a convenient resource if doctors were pressed to explain what was the matter. This pedantic method was then carried to such extreme, that it necessitates caution in referring to the writers of that time. Thus, in Dr. Churchill's comprehensive work on Diseases of Women (ch. vi.) he says that "Rheumatism of the uterus has been but slightly noticed in these countries; it is mentioned as long ago as 1685, by Dr. Charleton, in his essay " Inquisitio de causis Catameniorum et

---

* "As certain trees bear fruit without producing flowers (though it is rare), so some women may become pregnant without any previous established flux."—B. *Wenckius, De Menstruo Sanguine,* 1679.

† Cyclopædia of Anatomy and Physiology, art. "Uterus."

Uteri rheumatismo."* This was in reality only a dissertation on leucorrhœa; "rheumatismus" being simply used to denote a defluxion.

In its modern acceptance, the term leucorrhœa simply means and accurately describes an exaggeration of that healthy secretion which has for its office the due lubrication of that mucous surface extending from the fundus of the uterus to the ostium of the vagina. The cavity of the womb and the canal of its cervix are furnished with secretive organs which in the latter situation are especially abundant. "It is within the limits of moderation to say that a well-developed virgin cervix uteri must contain at least ten thousand mucous follicles."† The product of the intra-uterine and cervical follicles is uniformly alkaline; a glairy homogeneous exudation bearing strong physical resemblance to the clear fluid of a raw egg, but far more tenacious. There is a continuous gentle stillicidium of this from the os uteri during health, but it is increased in proportion to any congestive influence that affects the lining structure of the organ. The vagina corresponds so closely to the skin and assumes its characters so nearly when long prolapsed, that it has even been proposed to consider it a part of the epiderm. Its epithelium is tabular, it produces sebaceous material and an acid secretion which increases on any local excitement. The relation between the alkaline uterine efflux and the acid vaginal secretion was first observed by M. Donné, was

---

* Fourth Edition, p. 505.
† Dr. Tyler Smith on Leucorrhœa, p. 26.

specially applied by Mr. Whitehead, and the various sources of the secretions elaborately demonstrated by Dr. Tyler Smith. It is possible that the process of neutralization (with the gaseous products liberated when acid and alkali are brought in contact) exercises a slight local sedative action, whilst the natural heat of the passage induces resorption of the fluid part of the secretions, so that in health there is little or no out-flow from the vulva; all that presents is an agglomeration of the débris of fat cells and epithelium. This may accumulate as foul rolls of white exudation (especially in uncleanly women), in which the microscope detects myriads of vibriones. Leucorrhœa represents an excess of the secretive functions thus referred to. The chemical reaction is identical with that observed in many other glandular structures, and largely illustrated in the changes produced by the action of the alkaline excretion of the liver on the acid egesta that pass from the stomach.

The terms acute and chronic leucorrhœa are of questionable accuracy. The increase of secretion corresponds very closely to simple flux in other secretive organs, or to excess of the skin's action. It is the secretion that marks the disorder, and from which the name is derived; and the application of the word "acute" may serve to distract attention from something of greater moment. This may be judged from the symptoms which Lisfranc describes as those attending acute leucorrhœa in its extreme form. "After some inappreciable cause an itching of the genitals occurs, extending to the uterus, with sense of weight and heat in the pelvis. The hypogastrium is tense and tender. The womb appears to weigh down on the perineum. There is a dragging sensation about the loins, and persistent desire to pass water. The pudendum is tumefied, and if the parts be very much swollen, the patient has difficulty in sitting. There is nausea, lassitude, and restlessness. On the third or fourth day, a clear glairy discharge escapes from the vagina." In such a case it is evident that leucorrhœa is as inappropriate for designating an evident condition of active congestion or incipient inflammation as it would be to accept the character of the sputa for diagnosis of bronchitis.

The various characters presented by the leucorrhœal discharge depend on many causes, but mainly upon its source; whether chiefly uterine or chiefly vaginal. It may be clear and glairy; and if the use of the speculum be necessary, there is found a clinging accumulation around the os, often difficult to clear away. Here the condition is usually that which De Graaf described as an exuberant action of the numerous follicles of the cervix; a view which has received confirmation from the researches of Dr. Tyler Smith.* And this elucidation is confirmatory of the relations which obtain throughout between order and disorder; for it traces the immediate efflux to that follicular development which has for its ordinary office the supply of a cervical plug of mucus at the beginning of pregnancy; so that

---

* On Leucorrhœa, p. 85.

the changes then taking place in the womb might not be interfered with by causes acting from without. Vaginal leucorrhœa, as it occurs in children and during pregnancy and in cases of occlusion, or where the uterus is absent (see case, p. 121), is of a definitely white colour, and only becomes transparent and glairy when there is considerable local irritation and its amount is very profuse. From my own observations I incline to believe that the leucorrhœal discharge, which so irritates the tender skin of the inside of the thighs, frequently met with in stout persons of gouty diathesis, and which sometimes induces intense pruritus in aged people, has its source in the vagina, almost exclusively.

Leucorrhœa may occur at any period of female life. The white discharge to which children are subject is often accompanied by local heat and tenderness; hence suspicions may arise in the mind of the mother, which need to be authoritatively set at rest. Local inspection, or if there be any corroborative circumstantial evidence, careful microscopic examination of the discharge, will decide the cause and nature of the show. As a rule this leucorrhœa of children occurs where some existing irritation is specially determined by local causes. Thus, in strumous children during dentition, or where there exists an irritable bladder with incontinence, or the presence of a calculus,—in cases of scarlatina, where the urinary secretion is scanty and strong, and in others where ascarides irritate, the child frequently rubs the itching part to such an extent that profuse leucorrhœal discharge ensues from the vulvo-vaginal glands. The treatment of these cases simply depends upon recognition of the original cause. The method of tying the child's hands, often pursued by nurses, is sheer barbarity, so long as the cause of irritation is not removed. Simple local discharge readily yields to a weak solution of nitrate of silver or acetate of lead with morphia; but the occurrence of leucorrhœa in growing children often affords an early clue, indicating a condition of constitutional irritability which requires to be carefully watched. At and beyond the age of puberty, and up to the climacteric period, leucorrhœa usually accompanies local disorders of place, function, or structure. In the range of active uterine life thus comprised, leucorrhœa is the trouble most frequently experienced. In the large majority it is of systemic origin, occurring in young single women. In such cases it would be equally indecorous and unprofessional unnecessarily to talk to illiterate girls about their wombs. In the adult, leucorrhœa becomes a disorder whenever the wearing of a cloth is recognised as necessary by the patient, but it may go on to such an extent as to constitute an exhaustive flux. Here the relaxed vagina, constantly filled with the fluid, sometimes acquires a soddened appearance, the cervix uteri assuming a squared shape in place of its rounded contour. This " chisel-shaped cervix" was so often presented in cases where digital or specular examination has been necessary, that I cannot doubt its frequency also in those common cases of profuse leucorrhœa where local investigation is not needed.

A persistence of colourless or white discharge continuing

for some days after each menstruation marks the simplest form of leucorrhœa, as found in the virgin. In their ignorance, young women often reckon this as part of the period, judging only from the time during which they are put to personal inconvenience. It is necessary in such cases, to question closely, or, in case of doubt, to see the cloths that have been worn; for such an important diagnosis as that between absolute menorrhagia and successive leucorrhœa should not be decided by the cursory observations patients may happen to have made.

In its second stage leucorrhœa continues throughout the inter-menstrual time, so that patients, as they phrase it, are "never free." The increased action is thorough; the uterine and vaginal secretory functions being equally exercised in excess of their appointed duty: this is the state in which patients most frequently come under notice.

A third condition of this discharge is one accompanied, throughout, with local symptoms. If the uterus be at fault, a continuous glairy efflux, stiffening the linen, and accompanied by more or less of absolute suffering, directs attention to its source. If there be flakes of curd-like discharge or continuous flow of opaque, creamy fluid, accompanied by severe local soreness, rather than pain; then the source of the trouble is probably vaginal.

The existence of local disease causing menorrhagia usually induces persistent leucorrhœa during the intervals. On the other hand, a white discharge gradually increasing in amount is often coincident with the commencement of amenorrhœa.

Women recognise this vicarious action, and often cite the persistent leucorrhœa as a sufficient explanation of the menstrual irregularity. Any sudden check of eruptive diseases, of eczema, of profuse perspirations, of the secretion of the milk, and of accustomed discharges from other mucous surfaces, has been held to account for the occurrence of a vicarious leucorrhœa; and writers whose books are still deservedly held in esteem, refer to the neglect of habitual bleedings[*] as an occasional cause. Conversely, sudden stoppage of profuse leucorrhœal discharge may be followed by general disorder; but the mischievous results which ensue are usually confined to the organs constituting the generative cycle.

A periodic colourless discharge recurring regularly each month, and continuing several days, without any intervening efflux, occasionally precedes the first establishment of the true menstrual discharge. It may happen in adult women (the menstrua alba) may occur throughout the period of lactation, being replaced by the true catamenial efflux when the child is weaned; or may mark the commencement of the change of life. The occasional occurrence of leucorrhœal discharge during the time of pregnancy and its temporary increase as each monthly term comes round, is of great physiological interest in reference to ovulation. Practically it only marks an excessive action of the vaginal glands, and may be regulated by gentle injections of weak vegetable

---

[*] Dr. Davis, Obstetric Medicine, p. 343.

astringents or the use of tannin suppositories. The douche apparatus should not be employed, as its continuous action may disturb the cervical plug. In exceptional instances the fluid discharge has an offensive odour, so extreme that the patient "is a misery to herself." The local use of a weak solution of permanganate of potass (Condy's fluid ℨj, water ℨiv) usually suffices to remove this grievous complication of pregnancy. There is a belief, especially prevalent in the fen-districts (where leucorrhœa is common), that the children of women troubled with "the whites" during pregnancy, are liable to suffer from water on the brain. In fact, the same existent hereditary scrofulous taint which is the cause of hydrocephalus, frequently determines the occurrence of ordinary leucorrhœal discharge; and the same conditions of climate under which scrofulous diseases are engendered, appear to especially induce leucorrhœa. Other hereditary taints, particularly those of gout and syphilis, have been recognised as predisposing to the local affection, when the individual health is in any way impaired. Whatever depresses the vital energy, or slowly and progressively diminishes that natural resistant power which we designate Tone, tends to induce leucorrhœa, especially in girls where growth as well as repair have to be provided for. Delicate young women of leuco-phlegmatic temperament following sedentary occupations in close rooms; and those who, either by necessity or choice, take a poor and innutritious diet, with little healthy exercise, and scant or injudicious clothing, are especially subject to leucorrhœa. Its occurrence is coincident with other manifestations of mischievous results from this unhealthy mode of life : (*a*) the digestion is depraved ; (*b*) the mental faculties are impaired ; (*c*) the nervous correlations are disturbed, so that (*a*) the appetite is destroyed (*b*) hysteria in some of its multiple forms occurs; or (*c*) one or other of the neuralgiæ so commonly attendant on chlorosis and nutritive depravation, compels the patient to seek medical advice.

The frequent coincidence of leucorrhœa with some form of deranged digestion was especially pointed out by Dr. Mackenzie.* In his tabular record of a hundred successive cases of uterine disorder, sixty-five were accompanied with leucorrhœa; and there was in each case some notable digestive derangement. In sixteen of these, leucorrhœa was the only local disorder; and in fourteen out of this number there were marked symptoms of gastro-hepatic derangement.

When hysteria is coincident with that profuse leucorrhœa to which women of strumous diathesis are especially liable, it occasionally assumes a form which induces suspicion of cerebral disease or mental disorder. The patient is of vivid intellect, delicate frame, and impressionable nature; she shrinks from direct replies to absolutely necessary questions with a power of fence sometimes amounting to equivocation; so that the fears of watchful friends about mental disease or disorder

---

* The Relations of Uterine to Constitutional Disorder.

may seem exaggerated. These cases demand thorough investigation; for the hereditary strumous taint carries with it elements of disease which become dangerous if deposition takes place in parts where continuous action is unavoidable; as in the lungs or brain. Struma may induce leucorrhœa, and profuse leucorrhœa may lead to hysteria. Hysteria, plus struma and leucorrhœa, with a morbid intellectual brilliancy sometimes in inverse ratio to the physical degeneration, marks a condition in which tubercular disease progresses with terrible rapidity. Hysterical women of this kind, suffering from exhaustive leucorrhœa, are ready dupes to charlatans of all kinds—medical, religious, mesmeric, and spiritualistic; and the ignorance of unscrupulous impostors has consigned to destruction many a woman whose life would have been preserved by early and judicious attention to simple physical derangements.

The sympathetic physical disorders, especially affecting the nervous system, which accompany the presence of chronic leucorrhœa, and which depend on the same debilitating cause, especially induce that character of pain which, from its sharpness and intensity, is usually called neuralgic. One form of this fugitive suffering is so frequently connected with profuse leucorrhœa that it demands particular attention. It is commonly known as "Infra-mammary Pain," occurs almost exclusively on the left side, and principally at the seventh intercostal space, as its designation indicates. It is undoubtedly a reflex or radiated sensation, and various views as to the method of its induction have been propounded.* It occurs exceptionally in men when greatly debilitated by over-strain of mental energy without that corresponding physical exercise requisite to maintain the balance of health. Its frequency in women suffering from profuse leucorrhœa is worthy of note. Of fifty cases (taken in order as they occurred), this infra-mammary pain was present in forty. In some it was the trouble which induced the patient to apply for relief; in others the pain had gradually supervened. In two cases leeches had been applied, and in three blisters had been placed on the side, evidently on the supposition that there was pleurisy. Eight of the cases were under 20 years of age; twenty-three between 20 and 30; nine between 30 and 40. Of the ten cases in which no infra-mammary pain accompanied the leucorrhœa, the discharge in seven was distinctly attributable to local causes.

The treatment of leucorrhœa necessarily involves a careful consideration of the wide range of causes already mentioned. Where direct local symptoms are sufficiently urgent to necessitate thorough physical examination, any detected disorder of place or structure must be remedied before the leucorrhœal discharge will cease. In many of these cases, as in that large majority where the trouble is of systemic origin, astringent local applications may suffice to check the immediate flux: but such a result is of little permanent advantage to the patient. The relapse, when local treatment is no longer used, fre-

---

* There is an excellent paper on the subject by Dr. Martin, in the British Medical Journal, Sept. 10, 1864.

quently exceeds the original disorder: so that the woman loses heart, and comes to consider her ailment as incurable.

The long-recognised value of tonic medicines in leucorrhœa of systemic origin is fortified by daily experience; but in these cases, the causes which have gradually reduced the physical tone until the supplementary aid of therapeutical remedies becomes essential, should be carefully investigated; so that the life may be more healthily ordered, and the woman previously placed in such conditions that the course of tonic treatment, when begun, may have a fair field for its operation. The preliminary administration of purgatives often effects such a salutary change, especially in women of sedentary habits, that the continuous use of aperients has been somewhat indiscriminately advised. The common result is, that the more medicine the patient takes the more she requires. When once the body has been thoroughly cleared of accumulated excreta, tonic remedies will suffice to maintain the natural action, without strong aperients.

Wherever leucorrhœa has been described, iron has always been emphatically recommended as the sheet-anchor in treatment. Preparations of iron have been in use for upwards of three thousand years, and the first recorded case of their employment is one where the scraped rust was administered for debility of the generative organs.*

The most elegant preparations and those most advisable in the

---

* The Story of Melampus and Iphicles.

majority of cases, are the citrate of iron with quinine, the scaled pyrophosphate (which, if well made, should dissolve readily, and form a bright solution), the saccharated carbonate, the syrups of the superphosphate and of the iodide of iron. Less palatable, but cheaper and more convenient for admixture, are the old tincture of the sesquichloride and the sulphate; the former with hydrochlorate of ammonia and chloric ether, has for years formed the staple medicine in my hospital practice; but the combination of sulphate of iron with sulphuric acid and sulphate of magnesia, is a favourite combination with many. The action of iron as a remedy in cases of profuse leucorrhœa varies to a remarkable extent. Where not suitable, or the patient has not been previously prepared, there soon ensue symptoms of discomfort, indicating the impropriety of its continuance. In cases where it agrees with the patient, the dose may often very greatly exceed that ordinarily given, with an advantage correspondingly great. Observing this, I was gradually led, by noticing the results of treatment, to entertain the belief that all mineral medicines obey the same law in their influence on the animal economy; that, just as mercury, antimony, arsenic, and lead can be pushed in augmented doses until the saturation of the system is marked by certain special symptoms, so large quantities of iron, zinc, and probably other metallic remedies, may be advantageously administered until symptoms ensue which denote that the full effect is attained. Thus, I frequently commence treatment by giving a drachm of the tincture of the sesquichloride, a scruple of the scaled pyrophosphate, or ten grains of the saccharated carbonate of iron three times a day. And I find that so soon as the leucorrhœa ceases in coincidence with improvement of the general health, then the dose may be diminished, and gradually withdrawn, for its effects begin to tell; just as the props used for shoring up a dilapidated house must be removed by degrees, until the renovated fabric can stand unsupported.

The natural chalybeate waters, drunk at the source, are very valuable in cases of leucorrhœa with debility, especially where it has ensued after long residence in a tropical climate. The waters of Tunbridge Wells once held a very high repute in these cases, as did those of the pure chalybeate spring in the Well Walk at Hampstead, which at one time were daily brought to London in flasks and delivered to the houses of customers. Where the bowels are irritable, the strong chalybeate springs of the Isle of Wight, (containing a proportion of alum with the iron,) are very useful, and have even been bottled for exportation. Throughout this country, and in many continental spas (especially at Spa itself) iron springs of more or less strength are found. The common country remedy of " forge water," to be drunk clear and at the smithy, is a practical application of the conditions ordinarily enjoined—for the water in which the irons have been quenched is only clear early in the morning; and the patient has to walk to and from the source.

In combination with iron, or given separately according to the varying symptoms that attend profuse leucorrhœa, various tonic remedies may be employed with great advantage. Quinine—the mineral acids—the pure vegetable bitters, and those which contain tannin—astringents, salines, and the aperient salts combined with gallic acid—the oxide of silver, the sulphate of zinc, and preparations containing strychnia, such as the extracts of nux vomica and ignatia amara, and the solution of strychnia in phosphoric acid—all have their respective value in suitable cases; but not one of them is generally applicable. Dr. Marshall Hall recommended ergot as a remedy, and in cases of extreme uterine torpidity with atony and leucorrhœa its efficacy might be judged from what has been said as to its use as an emmenagogue (p. 123). In strumous cases, iodine and cod-liver oil are of notable service; the combination of phosphoric acid with tincture and syrup of orange being an excellent vehicle for the oil. The employment of vaginal injections in cases of leucorrhœa is of very ancient date. The modern syringe is little altered from that used centuries ago, but the uncouth douche apparatus, in effect a bladder and pipe, has been entirely superseded by more effective and more compact contrivances. Where it is required that the direct action of a drug shall be locally exercised, a syringe of glass or vulcanite used by the woman whilst resting in the supine position insures prolonged application of the solution. For this purpose lotions of acetate of lead or zinc, of sulphate of zinc or iron, of tannin and alum, of perchloride of iron, and of nitrate of silver are variously employed, but the last of these should only be applied by an experienced person. The purpose of the douche is to insure the passage of a free current of plain or medicated fluid across the surface whence the discharge proceeds, producing a tonic influence when cold water is used, and acting medicinally when camphor, opium, astringents, &c. are mixed with the fluid used. The best apparatus where an attendant assists is that of the ball and tube originally devised by Dr. Evory Kennedy, but it is often irksome when used by the patient. The long bags and other contrivances which act by gravitation are somewhat cumbersome, and I think inferior to the ingenious automatic "irrigateur" of Monsieur Eguisier. At least a pint of fluid should be used at each sitting. One of the most valuable hygienic appliances in the treatment of simple chronic leucorrhœa is the hip bath, as cold as it can comfortably be borne, and gradually extending the time of its use from a mere dip to ten or fifteen minutes. Natural sea water, or that artificially made with Tidman's salt, may be used with advantage in many cases. In general it is more serviceable taken in the forenoon than, (as is usually done,) on first rising in the morning. Sea-bathing and the use of baths of natural mineral waters, owe much of their special efficacy to the entire change of air, of life, and of habits involved, when patients resort to their use, and this comprises the secret of the advantage occasionally obtained under hydropathic treatment.

STERILITY represents disorder of the highest function of the organs constituting the female generative cycle. It may occur in perfectly healthy women suitably and happily mated, who have never suffered from any local trouble, and where no error of position, development, or action can be detected. Here it would be utterly wrong, in every sense, to sanction any operative procedure being attempted. Such interference is only justifiable where some remediable organic defect can be clearly made out. There is no such thing as an operation for sterility: nor is it possible to say that the removal of any recognised impediment will be certainly followed by impregnation.

Sterility may be Systemic, Ovarian, or Uterine. 1. Under the first head are included some most important physiological points, in reference to admixture and deterioration of race. So far as concerns the individual woman, it may be generally stated that all those conditions noticed as inducing systemic amenorrhœa (p. 114) afford, *à fortiori*, reason sufficient to explain accompanying sterility. Menstruation is a tentative process; and the probabilities of child-bearing are proportionate to the healthy accomplishment of this process previous to marriage.

2. *In Sterility of ovarian origin* there may be congenital deficiency, inefficient development, or recurring symptoms of ovarian dysmenorrhœa sufficient to account for the defect of procreation, as already described. Here the treatment has to be directed to the subdual of a condition of oophoritis or ovarian irritation; which may be a cause or only a coincidence.

3. *Sterility of uterine origin.*—An impermeable condition of

the Fallopian tubes has been described as a source of sterility, and attempts have even been made to overcome such supposed obstructions; but the proceeding is fraught with hazard. The body of the uterus is rarely at fault. Where constriction of the canal of the cervix is present, there is usually some accompanying history of foregone dysmenorrhœa of the obstructive kind. Great force from within (representing true expulsive effort) might overcome the difficulty after many pains; but the stricture may be absolutely impermeable so far as concerns impregnation, in that a barrier exists between the spermatic fluid and the extruded ovum. Such a constriction may occur in any part of the cervical canal. It may be at the internal os (usually from foregone flexion), in the course of the passage (as after injury during parturition), or at the external os (usually congenital or from previous erosion or ulcer of the lips). Where the stricture is at the internal os the conditions referred to when considering anteflexions of the uterus may supply a clue; for the long doubling together induces defective development of that part where the fold occurs.

Constrictions in the course of the canal are, I have reason to believe, more frequent than is usually credited. There may be the history of healthy maidenhood and of fruitful marriage, but, after parturition, the patient, on recurrence of menstruation, begins for the first time to suffer from dysmenorrhœa; and is thenceforth infecund. Such an obstruction may be readily recognised with the uterine sound.

Occlusion of the external os presents no difficulty in diagnosis. There is no doubt that a considerable number of erosions, &c. round the margin of the os are healed by the simple use of ordinary injections; sometimes even by mere rest and relief from local irritation. The cicatrization thus effected may induce partial closure of the orifice of the canal, or the same result may follow the injudicious use of caustics.* It is indisputable that dilatation or division of the canal of the cervix has in many cases given permanent relief to the dysmenorrhœa, and been followed by the result for which the patient was solicitous. But as in the majority of cases the constriction occupies only a small part of the passage, it is evident that division of the canal throughout the whole of its length is unnecessary, and attended with risk, since healthy structure is thus extensively cut. This constitutes an objection to the hysterotomes in general use, and probably explains the severe hæmorrhages which sometimes ensue. The instrument represented on p. 186 so far obviates this difficulty that it permits division of the constriction (previously diagnosed by the sound) without injuring the adjacent healthy tissues. After the operation the patient should be kept absolutely quiet for a while; since there is some risk of serious inflammation following, as in all cases where operations are performed on the uterine structures. A tent

---

* "Quibusdam post abortum uteri os exulceratur ac deinceps ad cicatricem perducitur, atque sic obturatio supervenit."—*Aëtius*, lib. xvi. ch. 51.

should be introduced after twelve hours to ensure continuous dilatation. I have never seen any bleeding follow this limited incision; but if it ensue the perchloride of iron is reported as successful for its arrest.

Where the constriction, in whatever part of the canal it may occur, cannot be distinctly traced to organic changes produced by those causes above enumerated, the simple use of dilating tents often proves successful. The ingenious instrument employed by Dr. Barnes[*] does away with the necessity for employing the speculum on their introduction. The laminaria tents are superior to those made of sponge, but necessitate some care, since they are more liable to expulsion on any effort. Sponge tents are preferable where it is required to so dilate the cervix that an examination of the cavity of the uterus may be made. For sponge itself really exercises very little direct power; merely soddening the parts in contact with it, so that they readily yield, but soon contract again. A string placed round an expanded sponge tent reduces it to its original dimensions without exercise of force; but the sea-tangle tent, when fully swelled out, resists this test of its power.

---

[*] Made by Messrs. Weiss, 59, Strand.

CHAPTER IV.

DISORDERS OF STRUCTURE.

MINUTE physiological investigation of the structures composing the human frame has afforded indubitable proof that the development of each tissue and organ, even in its immature or rudimentary stage, is ordered with special regard to an ultimate thorough fulfilment of its highest functional purpose. The nutritive activity which predetermines the order of development in different parts, has relation to the duties which each will have to fulfil. Thus, the lungs and larynx of the fœtus, absolutely useless organs during intra-uterine existence, are yet so completely finished before birth that the baby breathes and cries on the moment of its entry into independent life. Thus it is that the ovary of the child teems with Graafian vesicles; though years must come and go before any one of these can assume the semblance of a purpose.* The virgin womb is, in its structure, but a homologue of the gravid uterus, and the increase occurring during pregnancy is only an orderly development of tissue. For each of the coarse

---

* So far as I know, it has never been ascertained that a germ has escaped from a follicle and entered the oviducts, except just at the commencement of puberty.—Grohe: Virchow's Archiv. 1862.

muscular fibres of the gravid uterus is but a filling in (that is, a completion of the purpose) of one of the fusiform fibrils which make up the dense structure of the unimpregnated organ. Such increase of the proper tissue of the gravid uterus may augment its weight from one ounce to three pounds. The capability represented by this marvellous structural change is conferred by that provisional recurrence of tissue-renovation effected at each menstrual period, and which has already been described (p. 105).

The natural structural changes which take place in the ovaries and uterus represent a significant difference in the order which governs throughout the accomplishment of their respective duties. The ripe Graafian vesicle has, prior to its extrusion, undergone a process of advanced cellular organization never found in those intra-stromal ovules which still remain embedded in the substance of the ovary. This change is something more than a mere increase of growth or size; it represents an advance towards a new condition. It is the earliest indication of an *heterogeneous* development. Under favourable conditions, it may be elaborated into a distinct vitality, and determine the production of a new life. Hence the early activity of ovarian development for ensuring the establishment of perfect order in the functional co-relations, on which so much depends. The changes that occur in the healthy uterus during pregnancy are exclusively *homogeneous*. The virgin womb is simply a rudimentary organ of which the development is stayed; but with a special vascular arrangement, adapted for the due supply, on any exigency, of material to carry out to the full its structural purpose. This condition of latent power in the unimpregnated uterus is in accordance with a law of the economy already frequently referred to; the provision of power being constantly in excess of apparent physiological requirements. Thus: the heart beating seventy times in the minute, has a constant power equal, on emergency, to double that action; the muscles of the leg, when simply lifting the weight of the foot, may, if a slip occur, be suddenly called on to resist a strain two hundred times greater than that just previously thrown upon them. In these instances, and in many others, each tissue is constantly in perfect repair; and we judge its power, not so much by what it does, as by what it is always capable of doing. If the life of the virgin uterus were similarly ordered, with a wall-structure sufficient to lodge a full-grown fœtus, the physical inconvenience which would result is obvious. Hence the development of the organ is arrested whilst yet in a rudimentary condition; but it is surrounded and penetrated by vessels peculiarly and exceptionally arranged to facilitate rapid progress of its growth, when occasion arises. These are the curled arteries ("capreolorum vitium instar eleganter intortæ," as Swammerdam describes and figures them), and the venous plexûs already mentioned (p. 37). I repeat that the changes which take place in the structure of the uterus during pregnancy represent simply a continuance of its growth until the organ attains that perfect development for which provision was distinctly made throughout the time of virgin life. This view is assuredly more in accordance with that exquisite orderly arrangement which governs all the processes of life, than the bewildering suggestions which accredited the uterus as a "miraculum naturæ"—a microcosm—an animal within an animal; an organ undergoing extreme and marvellous changes, and such as to prohibit its consideration as merely an illustration of ordinary processes of nutritive development.

The practical applications of the distinctions thus drawn between ovarian and uterine purpose (a),—and considerations as to the important bearing which the order of uterine changes holds to certain modern views about its disorders (β),—may, more conveniently, succeed a mention of the proposed synopsis of diseases resulting from structural disorder.

1. CACOPLASIA.—Structural disease which is of systemic origin, where the blood itself is depraved and induces a resultant local disorganization—as in cancer and tubercle.

2. HETEROPLASIA.—Structural disease by which products in themselves natural, are developed in incongruent situations—as the hair and teeth in dermoid ovarian tumours.

3. HYPERPLASIA.
4. APLASIA.
{ Excess or deficiency in the reinstatement of particular component tissues, as in fibrous tumours and ulceration.

The above division accords pretty closely with the order adopted in the previous chapter. Thus cacoplastic changes are of systemic origin. Heteroplastic developments principally affect the ovaries. Hyper- and a- plasiæ represent changes which chiefly occur in the uterus.

a. It may be here premised that the structural disorders thus specially referred to the ovaries and uterus, indicate a remarkable analogy, in the method of their production, with the order described as governing healthy changes in these dominant organs. Setting aside the ordinary results which ensue from mechanical influence, from congestion and from true inflammation, the most serious and most frequent instances in which there is profound structural disorder are—1, cases of cystic disease of the ovaries (the most common form of "ovarian tumour"), and 2, accumulations of that elementary tissue which constitutes the bulk of the undeveloped uterus (fibrous tumours of the womb). In the first the products are heterologous: there is a chaotic generation of the identical materials which would have resulted on a natural continuance of the changes already commenced in each matured Graafian vesicle. It is in the uterus that hyperplastic changes chiefly occur—and these represent only an exaggeration of the nutritive changes especially provided for by the peculiar arrangements of the vascular supply. These relations will find further illustration when the hetero- and hyper-plastic changes come to be severally considered. They are here prematurely mentioned because of their relation to the distinctions already drawn between the purposes assigned to the ovaries and uterus, in carrying out the duties respectively assigned to the organs composing the female generative cycle.

β. Before considering in detail the structural changes comprised in the above synopsis it is necessary to make some reference to a much-vexed question especially important in the bearing which it has on the treatment of uterine disease. The decided opinions expressed as to the great frequency with which true inflammation and consequent ulceration affect the cervix uteri have been chiefly remarkable because of the large variety of disorders, general and local, held to thus find a common explanation. It is hardly too much to say that almost every ailment which could affect the frame of a woman has been directly or indirectly assigned a significant relation to some occult condition of uterine inflammation.

When my attention was first specially directed to diseases of women the controversy on this subject was at its height. The duty imposed on me necessitated the treatment, every year, of some thousands of cases of uterine disorder and disease. For the conscientious fulfilment of this responsible charge I eagerly sought every guidance, and the broad theory of the constant presence of inflammation and ulceration, with the consequent invariable necessity for local treatment in order to effect a cure, attracted especial attention. The opinion I then formed has been strengthened by many years of close observation among patients in every grade of life, and under every variety of conditions.

That true inflammation of the uterus occurs, and may affect any part of it, is of course indisputable; but it is a rare and grave affection. Its importance was dwelt on at great length by Aëtius, who even mentioned as one of the results of taking strong aperients that "there is danger lest from the vehemence of medicines of this sort (uterine) inflammation, ulceration, and fevers arise." His description is so graphic and concise that it is here appended, since I do not find that it has ever been translated.*

As error is said to be truth in the making, so the doctrines of Broussais, utterly fallacious when read by the light of modern pathology, indirectly led to a more precise study of the phenomena constituting true inflammation. As the word was then commonly employed it included everything and meant

---

* Inflammation of the uterus occurs from many causes. For it is set up by a wound, by suppression of the menses and abortion, by ulceration, by excessive coitus, by the pressure of a hard stool, by long and continued walking, by cold and by flatulence. Burning pains of the parts of women indicate it, of the pubes, of the bottom of the belly, and of the loins. And if the finger be introduced to the os uteri it feels to the touch hard, closed, hot and retracted, especially if the inflammation be within it or in the neck. For when the cavity or fundus of the uterus is inflamed the pain of the bottom of the belly indicates it, so that it does not admit any pressure externally, and especially the uterus is retracted at the inflamed part; on account of this cause its mouth and neck is turned away. But it differs from those (cases) mentioned as retraction of the uterus, because in inflammation the fever is acute, and the burning intense. But if the posterior part (of the uterus) has been inflamed, the pain more affects the parts around the spine, and the fæces are detained by the rectum being compressed. But when the anterior part is inflamed, dysuria or dribbling of the urine follows, from the bladder being pressed on, especially when the pain affects the pubes. But when the inflammation affects the lateral parts, the groins are swollen, and the thighs are heavy and moved with difficulty. But when the inflammation becomes more severe, symptoms of fever come on, disorder of the stomach through sympathy, swelling of the lower belly, burning, distension, weight of the coxæ of the loins, of the præcordia, of the groins, of the thighs; shiverings, diffused and pungent numbness of the feet, coldness of the knees, cold sweats of the extremities, small pulse, and death. But during its progress there is also vomiting, pain of the tendon of the neck, of the jaws, and of the forehead, especially at the base of the eyes. The urine and fæces are suppressed; and the inflammation being yet more augmented, the symptoms of fever increase, they become delirious, and grind with their teeth," &c.—*Aëtius*, lib. xvi. ch. 83.

nothing. Broussais dogmatized on what he saw. There was the positive presence of engorgement in the stomach and duodenum. He chose to attribute this to foregone inflammation, and to refer to this same cause many diseases then occult, but now thoroughly understood. His teaching was undoubtedly mischievous. The magic word inflammation solved every difficulty, and depletion was the universal remedy. Dr. Beaumont laid the axe at the root of this irrational theory, which prevailed long after the death of Broussais. He absolutely demonstrated that a condition of almost livid vascularity of the stomach is a physiological phenomenon which naturally attends the accomplishment of each process of digestion; and subsequent researches have shown that those diseases which Broussais unhesitatingly referred to gastric inflammation, notably fevers, had no such origin. Furthermore, the minute observations of exact pathologists have gradually given precision to the meaning of the term inflammation, and so defined the phenomena which attend its course as to permit a more accurate distinction in practice—where it was most needed.

The vascular relations of the stomach and uterus have in common a special arrangement for assuring immediate determination of a large supply of blood to meet functional exigencies. The elimination of some twenty pints of gastric fluid each day, with a continuous reparation of tissue, represents the offices subserved in the stomach. In the uterus the duties are, physiologically, of much the same kind; allowing for the difference between a vascular demand exercised many times each day, and one which has its efficiency tested only once a month, whilst the full operation of its ordained duties is only attained when pregnancy begins. In organs where the vascular supply is thus exceptionally arranged, it is notably important to mark accurately the boundary line distinguishing a determination of blood occurring in response to local irritation, from the phenomena that mark the occurrence of true inflammation. " The ' determination of blood to a part' here noticed, characterized by dilatation of the arteries, with increased flow of blood through the capillaries, must be distinguished from the ' congestion of inflammation' characterized by the accumulation and stagnation of red and white corpuscles in the vessels, tending to be abnormally adherent to each other and to the vessels. Mere determination of blood becomes obliterated after death by the post mortem contractions of the arteries, whereas the congestion of inflammation is persistent. It is an evidence of organic lesions declaring itself as distinctly in the dead as in the living; and thus the most important, if not the only sign of the early stage of inflammation having occurred during life is recognisable on dissection."* The most thorough upholder of the doctrine that uterine inflammation is of constant occurrence thus states his views on this point: "Mere congestion and inflammation appear to leave but little trace of their existence in the cervical mucous membrane. The changes that take place in the capillary circulation

---

* The Science and Practice of Medicine, by William Aitkin, M.D. 1863.

after death evidently remove or modify in part the alterations produced by inflammation in the mucous membrane perceptible to the eye during life."* If the point at issue involved nothing more than a pathological theory, the evident discrepancy here noted would be of minor interest. But the whole system of treatment in the majority of cases where the uterus is held to be in fault depends upon a due estimation of the value of this theory about the overwhelming frequency of uterine inflammation at all ages and in all conditions of life.

If it be accurate, then local treatment is always absolutely indicated, and there is no necessity to concern ourselves about the general health and the correlative influences which arise when any important organ is thrown out of order. Then no word can be said against frequent leeching, the application of strong caustics or of the actual cautery, with constant introduction of the speculum to allow of their use. The justifiable condition of nervous dread into which a patient falls when she hears of internal inflammation as constituting a part of her existence, would have to be particularly cherished. And thus narrowing our views of the true story of those pathological changes to which the uterus is liable, we might come eventually to adopt refinements such as that suggested by Scanzoni (one of the latest authorities in the school of special pathologists), who advises the dropping of melted sealing-wax on the cervix uteri

---

* On Inflammation of the Uterus, by Dr. Bennet. 1861.

as a valuable resource in treatment! I do not doubt that the appearances described and accredited to the presence of inflammation of the cervix uteri have been most carefully observed and faithfully recorded, for I have seen similar conditions in hundreds of cases. In the very large majority of these, the use of the speculum was necessary for diagnosis, the subsequent treatment being directed to the source of disorder. The method of treatment was in accordance with that principle already laid down (p. 79). The stages of disorder being carefully traced, endeavour was made to work back through the same series of conditions, reversing the action of those influences which induced the change from order to disorder, and from disorder to disease. Where physiology and pathology so closely touch that the teachings of either require to be constantly tested by information derived from the sister science, it becomes a matter of grave practical importance that every point be thus carefully weighed. It is clear that the diagnosis of inflammation, where there exists only such congestive condition as Dr. Aitkin so well describes, would simply tend to confuse; and to disturb the landmarks of scientific pathology.

There is yet a further argument against the theory of uterine inflammation being of such frequent occurrence that it would appear impossible for any woman to escape it. The orderly arrangement of the uterine vascular supply has been mentioned as representing perfect adaptation of means to an end. That this most exquisite physiological co-aptation should have been adjusted with utter disregard to the inflammation assumed to result from every slight disturbance, is not only contrary to the faith that is in us, but is opposed to the knowledge derived from study of other parts. Every highly vitalized organ undergoes recurring congestions—notably the lungs, the liver, and the kidneys. In bygone times these were generally treated by heavy bleedings. Under a wiser appreciation of the causes of disorder we now seek for and remove the source of obstruction.

The occurrence of ulceration of the womb has been very generally referred to a foregone state of inflammation. From what has already been mentioned it is evident that those very conditions adapted to insure the maintenance of uterine nutrition would become agents of structural disorder where the balance of the circulation is disturbed. Now the exoteric causes, whether mechanical or physical, by which this vascular equipoise undergoes derangement, are many and frequent, the uterus itself being only a passive agent. Thus, in cases of extreme prolapsus, there is generally present a superficial erosion of the mucous membrane around the os—whilst the adjacent parts are pale, dry, cool, and not tender to the touch. This may be called an ulcer, just as a bedsore may be so designated; but practically the history of such cases and the rational method of cure depends upon conditions with which true inflammation has certainly nothing in common.

Reference has already been made (p. 149), to a disordered textural condition of the uterus, which may be the forerunner of local complaints, both of place, function, and structure. Pathologically, it closely corresponds with that state of the heart-structure so admirably described by Dr. Richard Quain, and commonly known as fatty degeneration. Reparation is inefficiently effected; that transitory state which naturally attends thorough renewal of tissue (as in the uterine involution following pregnancy), becomes the ordinary condition of the organ. Those less considerable reparative changes which attend each menstrual period are equally defective. Happily there is no such necessity for constant action as exists in the heart: and, therefore, it is only when there ensue the results already noticed, as following on this defect in textural reparation, that the disorder is recognised. Due renovation of uterine structure requires that the general nutrition be in a healthy condition. If this be below par, the structure of the womb may just remain in a state which denotes arrest of the reparative changes; and with only negative results. As the fat and flabby heart represents a state of deficient renovation due to ineffective nutritive action, so the uterus, large, weak, and inactive, indicates deficiency of systemic power; and the general symptoms are explained by a condition only brought under notice by ensuance of one or other of those local disorders already mentioned. The patient may eat well, but what she takes is not turned to good account. She may be very plump, and appear the picture of health; but her muscles are flabby, the heart has to labour when unwonted exertion in the least degree accelerates the current of the blood, there is deficiency of power and of tone in every organ and structure; and the deposition of fat which plumps out the frame is rather an evidence of defective action than a sign of healthy condition. But there is an opposite physical state, no less important, where food, if taken at all, is not properly assimilated; where reparation is not effected because the conditions which ensure due renewal of tissue are not fulfilled. In these cases the women are thin, and worn, and weakly. The bruise which would produce no mark in a healthy person leaves on them a discoloration for weeks. There is little energy for effort, but there is still less power to repair the wear and tear which effort implies.—Here, also, the tissues which especially require continuous exercise of the reparative powers are those which chiefly afford direct evidence of mal-nutrition.

CACOPLASIA.—*An Absolutely Abnormal Structural Condition the Result of Unhealthy Constitutional Influences.*—Whenever the blood is vitiated, there ensues, sooner or later, some local manifestation of its disordered state. That part first succumbs which has least power of resistance; it may be congenitally defective, may be organically enfeebled by use or abuse, may be weakened by previous diseases, or rendered inordinately susceptible through peculiarities of its vascular arrangement. Certain of these blood changes can be readily detected; as in the rough physical tests formerly relied on for distinguishing inflammation, in the chemical process by which excess of urea is ascertained, and in the microscopical demonstration of a leukæmic condition. Other and more subtle poisons (as that of hydrophobia) have hitherto baffled all research: in this latter class must be provisionally included cancer, tubercle, and syphilis—diseases certainly due to attainted blood; whether the poison be hereditary, developed, or acquired, and these three comprise almost exclusively the cacoplastic changes which implicate the organs constituting the Female Generative Cycle. What induces the first occurrence of Cancer is utterly unknown, frequently some *hereditary* taint may be traced, but even this must at some time have had a beginning. Tubercle is usually *developed*, in whatever part the deposition occurs; and there is almost constantly some clear evidence of previous ill-health. Syphilis is generally an *acquired* disease, but in the majority of cases where it implicates the uterus or influences the function of the generative organs there has been a previous absorption of the virus and a resulting intermediate stage of blood poisoning.

CANCER.—The generally received opinion as to its hereditary nature is not borne out by the statistics of uterine cancer. An hereditary taint was traced by Lebert in one case out of seven (102 cases); by West and Paget in one out of six (199 cases); by Tanner in one out of thirteen (92 cases). It must be remembered, however, that the knowledge of the patient is usually imperfect; that a child is seldom told what disease has affected its parents; and that a considerable number of cases of cancer, implicating the stomach, liver, kidneys, brain, &c., are not diagnosed during life, nor is any post-mortem examination made. Moreover, the parent may transmit the germs of disease, yet die before the individual constitutional taint manifests itself. In one instance, the daughter (aged 30) died of uterine cancer, and the mother subsequently presented the first signs of mammary scirrhus. In accordance with a common belief, she considered that she had " caught the cancer" whilst tending her daughter.

Notwithstanding these difficulties there has been obtained evidence that in 83 cases of cancer, taken in order, one or other of the parents had similarly suffered in 45 instances.*

The organs which ordinarily exist in a state of latent activity, having special vascular provisions for ensuring rapid structural development or for sudden exaltation of functional action, are notably those in which cancer most frequently occurs. The uterus, the stomach, and the female breast, exist under such conditions, and it is in these that cancer most frequently occurs. In 9118 cases (including both sexes), collected by M. Tanchou from official sources, and where the disease occurred in 81 different situations, the organs above mentioned were implicated in the following proportions:— Uterus, 2996 cases; stomach and intestinal canal, 2670; breast, 1176.

The cervix is primarily affected in 97 per cent. of all cases of uterine cancer. The frequency of its occurrence coincides with the years of chief functional activity of the organ: thus, in 595 cases the earliest age was 25, and between 30 and 50 the numbers were as three to one of the cases occurring later in life. Uterine cancer is most frequent in fertile women (about 98 per cent.) and especially occurs in multiparæ; 69 per cent. of the cases having been pregnant more than four times.† Dr.

---

* Bartholomew's Hospital Reports, vol. ii. 1866.

† These calculations are deduced from statistics afforded by Dr. West, in his work on Diseases of Women.

Tanner gives a still higher average, 85·8 per cent., where the number of children exceeded six.

The practical deduction from these figures is one of serious importance. Cancer of the uterus runs its course more rapidly and is usually attended with more personal misery than is experienced when other parts are seats of the disease. No more deplorable human condition can be conceived than that of a sensitive woman, racked with incessant and agonizing pain, nauseated by the horrible fœtor of the continuous discharge, and with bladder and rectum perforated by the cancer.

However strong may be the hereditary taint it is clear that the virgin uterus is very rarely if ever attacked with the disease. But when once the functional activity of the organ is thoroughly aroused, a special susceptibility is induced; the local manifestation being especially determined to the cervix by those mechanical causes which affect this part of the uterus. And it is a grave consideration (remembering the utter inefficiency of treatment in checking the progress of true uterine cancer) whether in cases where an hereditary blood taint is recognised, it be not a duty to advise that the patient should not subject herself to the risks which matrimony would involve.

True cancer of the uterus is that which presents the characters of the medullary or encephaloid form. The other forms of malignant or cancroid diseases,—which are to some extent amenable to treatment,—require to be distinguished with the utmost care; for, in these latter cases, advantage may often be attained by local treatment, operative or otherwise; whereas in the more serious and more common form, any interference appears rather to accelerate the progress of the disease. That structural infiltration which in the medullary form of uterine cancer causes the surface of the cervix to feel hard, dense and irregular, or, in a more advanced stage, like banded gristly granulations which break down and bleed on being touched, led to a confused adoption of the term scirrhus as descriptive of every condition in which induration occurs. The distinction was very accurately marked by Aëtius.* That sensation of hardness which attends the first stage of true uterine cancer is not to be distinguished by physical characters from simple induration, and any expressed diagnosis should be scrupulously guarded. The remarkable rigidity of the parts around the uterus in cases of cancer, rendering the organ almost immobile, is very significant, when superadded to induration, nodulation, and frequent lancinating pains. If, in addition to these physical signs there occurs a sanious discharge, with occasional sudden and severe hæmorrhage, the prognosis becomes still less doubtful; but enlargement of the uterus with similar nodulation of the cervix occasionally occurs in plethoric women about the change of life, often accompanied by sharp attacks of menorrhagia and sometimes with that uneven and nodular cervix left after difficult labours. The next succeeding symptoms of

---

* Of the indurated cervix he says, "Duritiæ itaque circa os et collum uteri consistentes facile curantur," ch. 84. Of uterine cancer he states, "Tumor circa os uteri reperitur durus, ad tactum renitens, inæqualis, eminens, colore fæculentus, ruber aut sublividus. Proinde affectio quidem hæc incurabilis est."

uterine cancer are unmistakeable; the peculiar odour which the discharge presents; the gnawing, burning pain; and the foul ulcer which gradually involves both the uterus and the adjacent organs—the bladder being usually that first implicated.

The continuous pain of cancer, usually worse at night, accounts in some measure for that worn and anxious look, which differs so widely from the facial expression noticed in consumption, where the emaciation is equally extreme. Moreover, the cancerous cachexia is usually accompanied by a peculiar and characteristic colour of the skin, very much resembling the tint of ordinary yellow soap. In rare instances there is entire immunity from pain. In one case under my own care, and where I had the advantage of Dr. Tyler Smith's opinion, there was little or no local suffering even to the end. The hæmorrhage that attends uterine cancer (often the earliest noticeable symptom) appears to depend on the same causes which induce local determination of blood in other conditions of structural disorder, as polypus &c. Hence the importance of immediate physical examination without waiting for arrest of the issue of blood.

The copious fœtid discharge of uterine cancer, at first thin, greenish and acrid, afterwards sanious or even black, with ragged flakes of disorganized structure, is usually proportionate in amount to the progress of the disease and the extent of destructive action. The odour is so characteristic and clinging that it may often be recognised on entering the patient's room. Every kind of offensive vaginal discharge has come under my notice, some of them even more pungent and loathsome than that accompanying cancer, but none with the enduring odour which the finger retains for hours despite of washing and disinfectants.*

Treatment.—Very considerable advance has been recently made in the direction to which our endeavours are, unhappily, limited. Much can be done to afford relief from suffering, and to ensure that euthanasia so ardently looked for by the patient. The disinfectant and deodorizing properties of Condy's fluid, duly diluted; of carbolic acid (which, with soda and spirit, affords a most valuable lotion); of the chloride of zinc solution, &c., have led to their common employment as injections in cases of uterine cancer. A lotion of bromine has been advantageously used by Dr. Wynn Williams. This important agent was first recommended by Landolfi, and its general value was investigated by Dr. Glover. I have employed it, both in solution and in the compound condition (as bromoform). Its influence is deodorant, and I believe that it checks in some degree the destructive action, and therefore equivalently relieves suffering. The strength advised is ten drops of bromine to the half-pint. I have used, with similar advantage, an injection of sulphate of tin, two grains to the

---

* An illustration of the peculiar persistence of the cancer smell, was afforded some years ago, when the plastered walls of the cancer ward in one of the London Hospitals had to be scraped previous to painting. Some of the workmen absolutely vomited from the stench given off when the plaster was disturbed; for its porous nature had caused it to absorb and retain the foul odours.

ounce. This remedy has also afforded great relief when applied (of the same strength) in cases of mammary cancer. Bags of charcoal, or of gypsum mixed with tar, applied to the vulva are useful for preventing the odour of uterine cancer being offensive either to the patient or her friends. The room in which she lies should have painted walls, be thoroughly ventilated, and basins of dilute Condy's fluid placed under the bed—to be renewed whenever a scum forms on the surface.

The hæmorrhage in cases of uterine cancer may be almost invariably checked by local application of dry solid perchloride of iron—a method evidently preferable to the use of less potent astringents, as alum, tannin, nitrate of silver, &c. The styptic colloid recently introduced by Dr. Richardson (a strong solution of tannin in collodion) may also prove of service as a local astringent in cases of cancer. Topical applications have an advantage over medicines administered by the mouth, such as the mineral acids, gallic acid, alum, opium, matico and lead &c.; since these tend to induce that constipation, which is always so troublesome a complication in cases of uterine cancer. The importance of selecting remedies which may alleviate pain without interfering with the due exercise of the ordinary functions of life is especially to be regarded in cases of cancer, where, sooner or later, sedatives will have to be constantly administered. Hence opium in the crude form is objectionable, because it produces costiveness, and chloroform cannot be used for long without inducing sickness. The hypodermic injection of solutions of morphia is one of the most valuable means of affording temporary relief from the pain of cancer—and the operation may be very continuously had recourse to, without any apparent ill-consequences. Injections per rectum of the liquor opii sedativus, or of solutions of morphia, have the advantage that the small ball and pipe can be used by the nurse or even by the patient herself. Indian hemp, hemlock, henbane, lettuce, and other sedatives, when given, as they must be, in very full doses, require that the special characteristics of each patient be considered in selecting the remedy. The tincture of hemp (with ammonia), the succus conii (with spirits of nitre), and lactucarium (with sulphuric ether), have appeared in certain cases to be more efficacious than morphia. That troublesome cutaneous irritation which occasionally ensues after the morphine salts may be obviated by combining a small quantity of James' powder with the sedative pill.

The General Treatment.—It is indubitably true that cancer, like other hereditary diseases, especially attacks those members of a family who are congenitally weakly, or whose vitality is diminished by an injudicious, or exhaustive mode of life. It follows that, when once any hereditary taint can be traced, the importance of carefully guarding the general health should be forcibly represented to the patient. I thoroughly believe that cancer, equally with tubercle, might be averted, if it could be absolutely assured that the standard of physical health should be constantly maintained. A person with hereditary tendency to disease of whatever kind dare not risk the continuance of functional disorder, since this is the vantage-ground from which disease starts. Tubercle will not be deposited in a well-inflated lung periodically filled with pure air, and through which the blood courses without check. The result of statistics concerning uterine cancer is quite as definite in demonstrating the absolute immunity of the virgin organ where its functions have been efficiently fulfilled.

Those other local diseases, recognised as of malignant type, which affect the ovaries or uterus, allow a broad line for distinction from the cancer above described. Their progress may be checked, the character of the disease may be modified by judicious treatment, and in some cases ovarian tumours, apparently consisting of colloid cancer, or distinctly epithelial outgrowths from the cervix uteri, have been removed without recurrence of the disease. Epithelioma and rodent ulcer are recognised as by far the most frequent of all these cancroid conditions of structural disorder.

Cauliflower excrescence, epithelioma, or epithelial cancer, is specially marked by coarse sprouting granulations, which protrude from the lower zone of the cervix uteri. The disease was first accurately distinguished by Dr. John Clarke, and admirably described by his brother, Sir C. M. Clarke. It is a morbid outgrowth, having on its irregular surface a glazy membrane, from which there is exuded a thin and subsequently sanious discharge rapidly increasing in quantity; the sanguineous element becoming more and more marked. It has been observed that the mushroom-like spread of the disease is very distinctive.* It expands like the uncompressed part of a champagne-cork, and the healthy upper zone of the cervix uteri may frequently be traced, if the finger is passed beyond the excrescent mass of disease.

Treatment of these epithelial out-growths by direct application of caustics has been fully tried, and the result is eminently discouraging; but absolute removal of the diseased mass with the écraseur (using the speculum of Dr. Marion Sims and the ether spray), with a subsequent free application of one or other of the potent caustics now in common use, appears to have prevented the recurrence of the disease in several well-authenticated instances. The actual or galvanic cautery, exsiccated sulphate of zinc, chloride of zinc, the pastes of arsenic, nitric acid, concentrated carbolic acid, acid nitrate of mercury, and the perchloride of iron used in a dry state, are the most useful applications after removal of the diseased out-growth.†

Rodent ulcer of the uterus, the corroding ulcer of Sir C. Clarke, is a destructive form of disease which has not as yet been traced to any distinct cause. It usually attacks the os uteri, but sometimes occurs in the vagina or at the external parts. There is an eating away of the surface by steady extension of ulceration without surrounding induration, and the progress of the disease frequently intermits. The uterus, even

---

* Dr. Braxton Hicks: Guy's Hospital Reports, 1866.
† The Modern Treatment of Cancerous Diseases by Caustics. By Langston Parker. 1867.

when extensively implicated, remains free and moveable, the disease not appearing to extend beyond the limits which it has attained at the time of examination. This form of ulceration has many points in common with lupus exedens, as regards its symptoms and progress, its pathology, and the results which attend that decided modification of tissue-changes induced by local application of potent caustics. The disease may be unaccompanied by pain (as in rare cases of true cancer), but there is usually that sensation of gnawing so characteristic of lupus—wolfish. Aëtius affords an equally characteristic reason for use of the same term.*

The treatment of corroding ulcer must be immediate and decided. Its good effect depends on a thorough destruction of the unhealthy surface; and the prognosis must be guarded until the results of this heroic method of modifying the nutritive changes can be determined. The same potent caustics which arrest the progress of lupus have been advantageously employed in this disease.

Tubercle.—The uterus may present local evidence of tubercular deposit in advanced stages of the general disease; but primary implication of the organ rarely if ever occurs. Those conditions of cervical disease which Lisfranc considered to be due to tubercular ulceration, and the circumscribed yellowish pustules referred by Kiwisch to the same condition, probably

---

* "Maleficum autem et ferum ulcus à feris ac malignis animalibus cognominatur; est enim protervum et curatione efferatur et manuum tractatione exacerbatur."—Lib. xvi. ch. 43.

depend on other causes—as pointed out by M. Robin and Dr. West. Attention has been recently directed to the coincident occurrence of erosion of the cervix uteri with advanced phthisis, and, indeed, some of the most distressing symptoms attributed to its presence. Such local structural disorder is most likely to occur wherever the constitution is debilitated and the reparative power diminished, during fecundity; but there is no evidence that the condition described has any special relation to tubercle, especially as the symptoms attributed to its presence occur with equal frequency in males.

In advanced phthisis, the lining structure of the body of the uterus occasionally undergoes tubercular degeneration, as proved by microscopic investigation. The organ is large and heavy, but freely moveable, and the cervix is rarely implicated. There is generally some functional disturbance and tenderness, with gradually increasing pain. The attendant leucorrhœa presents an occasional admixture of flakes and shreds of the disorganized tissue. These cases are distinguished from cancer by the physical characteristics of the uterus, by the marked constitutional disease, by the absence of hæmorrhage and of fœtor. Recent pathological observations of extirpated ovarian tumours appear to indicate that true tubercular deposition may accompany, even if it does not sometimes determine, the occurrence of the disease.

Syphilis.—Where the syphilitic poison has come to infect the whole mass of the blood, and where the woman becomes unhappily pregnant, the disease appears to be specially determined to the reproductive organs. Sometimes its influence is manifested by recurring abortions; in others, the offspring afford unmistakeable indications of the specifically unwholesome state of the parent. In one instance under my care, a woman, already three months pregnant, was then infected by her husband. The primary vulvar sore and syphilitic tubercles of labia soon yielded to iodide of silver applied in the nascent condition.* Iodide of iron was given internally. Here the child appeared and continued perfectly healthy, as though the disease had been arrested before any infection of the blood had occurred. In other cases, even where every trace of the syphilitic disease appears to have been eradicated in both parents, the offspring afford indubitable evidence that the lingering hereditary taint still remains. The influence of constitutional syphilis in inducing disorder of uterine structure is not so clearly recognisable. Mr. Acton says, " In women who suffer from syphilis in its worst form in all other parts of the body, the os uteri is very seldom affected."† Mr. Whitehead considers that endo-cervical irritation, a mottled and patchy appearance of the cervix, aphthæ and warty growths, are often evidences of constitutional syphilis. There is one appearance of the uterine ulcer which has appeared to me sufficiently distinctive to deserve special attention (*see* Aplasia), and which I conceive to be attributable to the poison lurking in the system of the

---

* As described in my paper on the Topical application of Silver Solutions: *Lancet*. 1865.

† On Diseases of Urinary and Generative Organs.

male having just influence sufficient to modify the characters of a cervical sore already existing, although not potent enough to affect an unbroken surface.

HETEROPLASIÆ.—Among the *curiosa medica* are recorded many instances where a child, or parts of a child, have been found within the body of another naturally born. In some cases, these monstrosities have remained without notable change until adult life, and only been discovered after death. They have occurred in both sexes. Hence the doctrine of congenital inclusion has been urged as sufficiently explaining the presence of those heteroplastic structures found in ovarian tumours. The occurrence of these organized products in independent cysts at one time evidently attached to an ovary— or in the uterus and bladder, after adhesions allowing the abnormal products to pass into the cavities of these organs—are of secondary importance to the determination of the conditions under which they were originally produced.

Ovariotomy implies such serious responsibility (since the only issue is to life or death, and the chance of life often depends on the skill of the surgeon), that the majority of cases are prudently referred to those operators who have had the largest experience. Their special interest in the subject has led to careful and skilful investigation into the nature and pathological characteristics of each tumour removed; and the observations thus made have advanced, with unexampled rapidity, the progress of ovarian pathology.

There is no reliable evidence that the development of teeth, the growth of hair, the production of cartilage, of true bone, or striped muscular fibre, and other heteroplastic substances within the ovaries, has ever been recognised until after puberty; whereas fœtal inclusions, elsewhere found, are usually recognised early in life. The doctrines of Meckel, Haller, Velpeau, and Cruveilhier (that these products result from disorders of impregnation, or from extra-uterine fœtation), are disproved by well-marked cases in which heteroplastic deposits were found in tumours removed from virgins.

There only remains the view already suggested (p. 214). It is believed that an inchoate germinal change attends the maturation of each Graafian body in a healthy ovary, prior to any influence exercised from without. This inherent power, stimulated to a higher degree of development, would induce those changes which have led recent industrious observers to consider that every heteroplastic deposition in dermoid cysts "represents an ovum which has undergone a certain amount of development—that it is a perverted attempt at parthenogenesis."*

HYPERPLASIA }
APLASIA. } These terms bear a distinct meaning, which appears to justify their use as descriptive of conditions where something beyond mere excess or deficiency of general nutritive action is involved. In hypertrophy there is a thorough increase of growth, each tissue retaining its relation with other parts of the limb or organ. All increase

---

* Ovarian Physiology and Pathology. By Dr. C. G. Ritchie. 1865.

alike; as in atrophy all the textures become proportionally wasted. In Hyperplasia there is an increased local determination of constructive material similar to that which initiates hypertrophy; but its usage (πλασις) is unequally distributed. In Aplasia there is defect in reinstatement of structure, certain tissues being specially affected. But there also occur structural disorders, presenting a clear history of gradual transition from excess or defect of development to a state which is one of actual disease.

From the ostium vaginæ to the fundus uteri the lining membrane is continuous; but its physical characters vary throughout. So also those structural changes which specially affect these lining tissues (as distinct from hyperplastic changes of stromal origin) present marked variations of character in accordance with the situation of their occurrence. The large and numerous vulvo-vaginal papillæ and those projecting folds to which they are chiefly attached often present this kind of outgrowth, which begins with simple hypertrophy, but readily passes on to a condition where the natural relations of form and structure no longer obtain. There may be simple villous prolongations, which shrivel and die when touched with a caustic; or the carunculæ may be so enlarged as to present an absolutely obstructive fringe of pedunculated polypoid growth, inducing continuous leucorrhœa and other inconveniences. These are readily removed with the écraseur, or by application of acid nitrate of mercury several times repeated. The troublesome warts (usually of specific origin), which occupy the same situations, may be successfully treated with the same potent caustic, or by touching with chromic acid.

Those painful vascular outgrowths from the female urethra, which cause such severe and varied suffering, are readily recognised by their local symptoms and appearance on examination. They yield to application of nitrate of mercury or of the dry perchloride of iron; but where the excrescence is unusually large, it is advisable to employ the wire écraseur of Wyld before applying the caustic. The pain caused by micturition in these cases sometimes induces the patient to delay emptying the bladder until it attains that extreme degree of distension which the capacity of the female pelvis specially allows. Such inordinate strain, whatever the cause, frequently induces subsequent cystic irritability, so that the inability to retain the urine may really be the most marked symptom. Small doses of tincture of lytta, the use of cold hip-baths, and strict injunctions to empty the bladder at stated intervals, will usually remedy this very troublesome condition. In married women, the severe suffering endured (sometimes causing much social unhappiness) is only relieved on removal of the urethral outgrowths. The intricately folded lining tissue of the canal of the cervix uteri is occasionally the seat of hyperplastic outgrowths, sometimes as vascular as those last mentioned. They may surround the os like a fringe of coarse granulations, denuded, soft, and readily bleeding when touched; or one or more may be attached high up within the canal. Such little vascular tumours are usually pedunculated, through the recurring expulsive efforts induced by their presence. On account of this continual urging in one direction, the growth may become gradually elongated, areolar structure being developed in the pedicle, so that the polypus may attain several inches in length. In such cases there is usually a coincident development of the follicles so profusely dotted amid the folds of the arbor vitæ, so that the protruding polypus may appear lobulated; each prominence representing an obstructed follicle which yields a clear tenacious fluid on being pricked. Sometimes obstruction of a follicle induces its gradual independent enlargement, producing a cystic tumour, which may attain the size of a large grape. Whether the hyperplastic growth be papillary, compound, or cystic, the symptoms are those produced by the presence of a foreign body distending the canal of the cervix—expulsive effort and forcing pain, with consequent uterine and bladder irritation; dysmenorrhœa, often menorrhagia, always sterility. Removal of the growths, either by caustics, the polypus forceps, or the écraseur, relieves the more urgent symptoms; but the sensitive vascular texture often retains its irritability, and remains congested for some time; a condition only to be gradually removed by attention to the general health, and especially by means which tend to relieve the local congestion and subdue the irritation—such as bromide of potassium, ammonia, Indian hemp, aconite, saline aperients, belladonna, and the cold douche or hip-bath. Within the cavity of the uterus the lining tissue occasionally gives origin to small flattened polypoid excrescences, and cystic growths, varying in size from a pea to a grape, may ensue from follicular obstruction. In one case where several such growths were present, they successively burst on being grasped with the forceps. The prominent vascular loops which characterise the lining structure of the uterus are necessarily liable to congestion, if there be any check to the free current of the circulation, and the prominence they assume when thus injected has led to their being mistaken for true villi. Such vascular turgescence differs in cause and character from true inflammation; and the term "endometritis," if used at all, should be very carefully restricted, since over-officious local interference in cases of simple congestion is very likely to produce inflammation.

The stroma of the cervix and body of the uterus (especially that of the posterior wall) may be simply hypertrophied and indurated; varying in extent from mere nodular outgrowth to such general enlargement of the body of the uterus that the shape, size, and direction of the organ becomes considerably modified. In the cervix there may be enlargement of either lip—sometimes so protruding as to overlie and conceal the canal—or nodular hypertrophy, simple or multiple, destroying its rounded contour. These projections, surrounding the os, and usually ensuing after a severe confinement, are sometimes so hard as to lead to the suspicion of cancer. Dr. Henry Bennett has pointed out the important distinction, that after laceration " the fissures which separate the lobes radiate round the cavity of the os as a centre—which is not the case in a cancerous tumour—each separate lobe being perfectly smooth in itself, and free from tubercles or superficial inequalities." In other cases the whole cervix may be greatly widened out without increase of length, or be so elongated (either conoid or digitate in shape) as to be visible on separating the labia.

Deficient involution, or undue uterine congestion whilst that process is going on; menstrual checks followed by active local determination; injury of the cervix, or other mechanical causes, often lead to such excess of growth. Here the abnormal enlargement remains long after the cause has been removed, frequently without undergoing further change. In one case a cervix as large as an orange had, by all accounts, existed without notable alteration for two years. It rapidly diminished under the local use of iodine, a plan of treatment remarkably efficacious in the majority of these cases. The iodised cotton recently introduced by Dr. Greenhalgh,* is a neat and cleanly method of insuring steady and continuous action of the remedy; the general treatment being of the kind already described as specially adapted to relieve an engorged uterus by unloading the portal system. Cases of simple hypertrophy indicate an excess of true growth; but in hyperplastic depositions there is inordinate development of one structural element, notably illustrated by the fatty tumours which occur in areolar structures. The

---

* Prepared by dissolving two ounces of iodide of potassium and one ounce of iodine in eight ounces of glycerine, saturating eight ounces of wool with the solution, and then carefully drying. A pledget (with a thread attached) is placed against the cervix.

much-questioned assertion of Bayle, that uterine fibrous tumours are to be found in one-fifth of all women who die after the age of thirty-five, probably originated from grouping together cases of hypertrophic enlargement and hyperplastic growth.

Fibrous Tumour and Polypus Uteri.—These closely allied growths are the most frequent of all organic disorders of the true uterine structure. In the beginning they represent simple increase of nutritive activity; it is only when the material thus supplied has its operation restricted to a small area, to the elaboration of one tissue and its continuous aggregation, that the term hyperplasia becomes applicable. In the majority of cases there is a corresponding development in those parts of the uterus not implicated by the new growth, even up to that muscular condition which obtains at the latter months of pregnancy. A shred of a fibrous tumour may be indistinguishable from a similar portion of the stroma of a healthy virgin uterus, as observed by many pathologists. But there is a notable difference between the tumour-structure, consisting of fusiform fibrils destitute of order and direction, inchoate, purposeless, and rolled together into an irregular mass, and the adjacent tissue of the same uterus, which has become simply developed through the flood of nutritive material determined to the organ under the impulse of the new growth.

Fibrous tumours formed in the substance of the uterine walls may so blend with the surrounding structure that it is difficult to distinguish any absolute line of demarcation; or the new growth may be so distinct that it can be readily shelled out from the adjacent parts. In the latter case, the tumour is often lobulated, whereas interstitial fibrous depositions usually follow the natural shape of the uterus. There may be several centres of deposit leading to the formation of independent tumours, all due to the same determining cause, but varying in the extent and rapidity of their growth, and the symptoms they produce. Multiple fibrous growths most frequently occur at the outer or sub-peritoneal surface of the uterus. The large single tumours, which occasionally attain such enormous magnitude (even equal to one half of the whole weight of the body), usually lie within the substance of the uterine tissue; and may be designated as intra-stromal fibrous growths. Those developed beneath the peritoneum (extra-uterine or sub-peritoneal), or produced at the inner surface of the womb (intra-uterine or sub-mucous fibroids passing into polypi), owe their distinction to mechanical rather than to structural differences. They are subjected to the influence of a continuous gentle movement in the adjacent parts, which increases as the growth of the tumour presents more decided resistance. Thus the peristaltic movement of the intestine, unfelt but constant, may induce gradual urging outward of any sub-peritoneal fibrous growth lying in the direction of their action. Such out-growths are occasionally found so pedunculated as to resemble a mushroom on its stalk; whilst in other cases the gradual extension of the pedicle leads to entire separation, and the roving tumour may take on a fresh attachment. In one instance which I had an opportunity of examining, the fibroma (about the size and shape of a kidney) had become fixed to the omentum. There was the history of an out-growth, moving with the uterus, having been diagnosed twenty years previously, of a severe fall followed by symptoms of peritoneal inflammation, with the subsequent recognition of a rounded tumour readily moveable and lying immediately beneath the abdominal parietes. This had been erroneously diagnosed as a moveable kidney; indicating the importance of thoroughly investigating all preceding symptoms. So far as my own research has extended, every case where a free fibrous tumour has been discovered within the abdominal cavity has occurred in the female sex.

The remarkable nodulosity which especially distinguishes growths from the outer surface of the uterus, probably owes this physical character in some degree to the moulding influence exercised by the never-resting action of the adjacent organs. This affects the out-growth only, and not the uterus proper. On the other hand, intra-stromal fibroma and intra-uterine polypi necessarily interfere with the action of the organ itself. The difference is of practical importance; for Cruveilhier observed, and Dr. McClintock has confirmed his opinion, that sub-peritoneal fibroids rarely produce uterine hæmorrhage; whilst those which project into the cavity of the uterus are invariably attended by excessive loss. These latter growths, occurring at the inner surface of the uterine stroma, soon become subjected to mechanical influence. For within the uterus there is a continuous unfelt urging peristaltic action, which is the physiological representative of expulsive effort. In health it serves to clear away accumulated secretions and to induce reparation of tissue. When developed to the utmost, there is called into co-operation the sympathetic action of other parts, and the uterus thus steadied and supported acquires that great direct power manifested in each labour pain. By a modification of the same force there is brought about the gradual pediculation and protrusion of an intra-uterine polypus.

The prognosis in cases of solid fibrous tumours, especially those developed in the substance of the uterine walls, has been considerably modified of late years; for reasons which I conceive to have an important practical bearing in reference to treatment. These hyperplastic growths chiefly occur during the years when the uterine tissue is most sensitive, and is kept in constant readiness to undergo the remarkable structural changes which accompany pregnancy. The fibrous tumour of the uterus has never been observed before puberty, nor is there any trustworthy evidence of its originating after the function of the uterus has entirely ceased. The rapid aggregation of the neoplastic structure during adult life, when once a nucleus has been deposited in the uterine walls, is sufficiently explained by those provisions already described as specially adapted for insuring a full supply of nutritive material to the uterus. The recent suggestion, that fibrous tumours of the uterus are often attributable to local determination caused by vicious habits is utterly unworthy of credit. Women suffering from this disease have already a sufficiently heavy burthen to bear without being subjected to suggestive cross-questionings, or to those suspicions which would naturally arise if the assumptions above referred to were worthy of any credit or consideration.

When the uterine function ceases, and the time of systemic change has passed, it has been noticed, especially of late years, that a corresponding alteration takes place in pre-existing fibrous tumours of the uterus. When, under the re-arrangement of the nutritive process, the free flow of plastic material is arrested, they sometimes simply cease to grow; but more frequently they gradually diminish in size, and may even entirely disappear. In rare cases there ensues a process of cystic degeneration, of purulent formation, or calcification. There have fallen under my notice ten cases in which fibrous tumours, originally large, have gradually dwindled after the climacteric period had passed; five were unmarried; three were barren wives; two had borne children, but in one of these the tumour first developed during widowhood. In two of the cases the patients had visited Kreuznach for several successive seasons. It follows, that the prognosis of a fibrous tumour developed after forty is more favourable than when it is formed earlier in life; and that whatever controls the local vascular determination will, *pro tanto*, arrest the growth of the tumour and liability to exhaustive menorrhagia or persistent uterine hæmorrhage: for the "tendency to death" in case of simple fibroma, is either from the pressure produced on adjacent viscera by the continuous growth, or from the exhaustive effects of recurring losses of blood.

The alterative influence exercised by iodine, bromine, and mercury has led to their extensive use of late years in the treatment of uterine fibroma; and the recorded results are very encouraging. Perhaps this is in some part due to the recent improvement in diagnosis of diseases of women, so that cases come under active treatment before the tumours have attained such magnitude as to produce mechanical obstruction. From the recorded histories, from inquiry, and from personal observations, I believe that the selection of the alterative administered is a matter of considerable importance. Where very profuse menstruation attends the development of uterine fibroid, and especially if it present the characters already described (p. 146) under the head of ovarian menorrhagia, the bromide of potassium with Indian hemp, in doses as large as can be borne, is indicated; continuing the bromide perseveringly. Where there can be traced any strumous or syphilitic taint, or if the patient be thin without absolute local suffering at the menstrual time, but with much leucorrhœal discharge, then iodine is most suitable, especially the iodides of ammonium and potassium with cod-liver oil.

When the woman is stout and with a thick layer of abdominal fat, the menstruation being natural or even deficient, and the tumour chiefly manifesting its presence by the local inconvenience, the mercurial treatment appears to be indicated. The periodide (Liq. hydrarg. perchlorid., ʒj; potassii iodidi, gr. iij; aquæ pimentæ, ʒvij; ter die) continued until the red line appears on the gums, and then perseveringly taken in diminishing doses, is that preparation which I have found most serviceable. One patient, æt. 34, continued its use for eight months, and the large nodular fibrous tumour became both less in size and softer in consistence. There is one important element in the treatment of fibrous tumours of the uterus which demands more attention than it has hitherto received. I refer to the regulation of the diet : the patient observing abstinence from gelatinous foods ; avoiding meat and beer ; partaking freely of fruit and green vegetables ; and drinking largely of any grateful diluent, in order to insure free elimination by the kidneys.

Where fibrous tumours attain to such size that inevitable death must follow any further increase, it is certainly right to submit the question of operation to the patient or her friends. The process of gouging the fibrous mass from within the uterus, and so setting up a disintegrative action involves a great amount of prolonged personal suffering, whilst the results hitherto obtained have not been encouraging. By gastrotomy it may be found possible to effect enucleation of the tumour, or, at the worst, to remove the whole organ—this has even been successfully accomplished. The dread of opening the peritoneal cavity has greatly diminished since the operation of ovariotomy has been revived with such marked success, and the precautions necessary to be adopted are so much better understood.

Polypus Uteri.—Rapidly recurring hæmorrhages so commonly attend the presence of uterine polypus, that they may be regarded as one of the most distinctive symptoms. The loss chiefly occurs when the neck of the uterus begins to undergo dilatation, or after the tumour has passed into the vagina. Where uterine fibroids encroach on the cavity, a somewhat similar mechanical force may be exercised on the upper part of the canal of the cervix; and it is in these cases, as already mentioned, that uterine hæmorrhage most frequently accompanies fibrous tumours. It is not unreasonable to suppose that the mechanical dilatation of the cervix, which Dr. Barnes has shown to be one of the most reliable methods of inducing expulsive action, may, if slowly effected by a comparatively hard substance, cause engorgement of the uterine tissue with resulting menorrhagia. On this view, the relief from hæmorrhage which follows division of the cervix in some cases of fibrous tumour, as observed by M. Nélaton, Mr. B. Brown, and Dr. McClintock, is readily explicable. "When hæmorrhages from the uterus arise from a polypus, medicines are useless. The only effectual way to cure the hæmorrhages is to remove the polypus." This dictum of Dr. Gooch admits of no exception. Whenever there is continuing uterine hæmorrhage, a careful local investigation should be instituted, and the way in which this is done is important. Women, naturally enough, often ask that the examination may be deferred until the flux has abated; but it is whilst the hæmorrhage is going on, when the uterus is low down, and the os patulous, that the diagnosis is most readily made. The recognition of polypus lying in the vagina may be attended with difficulty, for sometimes there is very close resemblance in shape and size to an irregularly hypertrophied cervix; one which I removed two years ago has a chink precisely corresponding to the os uteri.

The diagnosis of intra-uterine polypi, can only be certainly made by dilatation of the external os, so that the finger may be introduced within the cavity of the womb; but a very important guide in these cases is often afforded by the condition of the os uteri itself, which is usually round and tense and thin if the polypus has entered the neck. With the patient well coiled up on the side, and one hand pressing on the hypogastrium, it is almost always possible in these cases to so dilate the opening, that the finger can pass on to distinguish the character of the intra-uterine growth. The removal of a polypus uteri which has passed the uterine neck, necessarily involves a consideration of the constituent materials of its pedicle. Recent pathological observation has demonstrated that this consists, with very few exceptions, of simple areolar structure, having a coating of mucous tissue. In the natural effort to extrude and entirely throw off the polypus, the vascular supply of the tumour has been gradually diminished, so that its surface readily degenerates, and may even present a sore which has the appearance of gangrene.

The application of a ligature around the neck of such a polypoid excrescence necessarily increases this evil. This method of treatment has been entirely superseded by operations which at once remove the tumour, without that slow process of sloughing which the ligature involved. It was formerly supposed that the hæmorrhage proceeded from the tumour itself; it is now clearly shown that the vascularity usually diminishes in proportion as the stalk of the tumour elongates, so that its final separation (as in the cases of extra-uterine polypi) is unattended with hæmorrhage. Some few cases are recorded where an artery of considerable size has been found in the pedicle; so it is always advisable, if possible, that the finger be passed round the tumour to ascertain the size, attachments, and vascularity of the pedicle.

When the pedicle of a vaginal polypus exceeds the thickness of the middle finger, it may be divided either with the écraseur, the polyptome, or by the use of curved scissors. The wire écraseur of Dr. Braxton Hicks is now very generally used, because of its ready application round the tumour. Dr. Marion Sims has introduced a most ingenious adaptation, by which he is enabled to readily grasp large intra-uterine polypi with the chain-écraseur. In ordinary cases, where the pedicle of the polypus is small, any long forceps, sufficiently strong to ensure a good grasp, will enable the removal of the tumour. My "speculum forceps" (p. 260), is specially arranged to admit of its being used for polypi, and I have several times removed tumours as large as a turkey's egg with this instrument alone. The method I usually employ in cases of true polypi lodged in the vagina, depends upon that readiness with which areolar structure, when thoroughly stretched, may be divided; just as a strained rope flies asunder at the touch of the knife. The tumour is firmly seized and drawn down, so that the fingers may pass it to touch the os. If the uterus is unaffected by torsion of the polypus, the pedicle usually gives way after two or three turns, and may at once be brought away. If the uterus move, it is probable that there is a short pedicle, with partial inversion. Then I serrate with a scalpel the nail of the left forefinger, and whilst the pedicle is on the stretch, saw it through with the jagged edge thus produced. The polyptome, which encircles and cuts through the pedicle, and the thimble with a curved projecting knife, are more complicated means of effecting the same end.

When the polypus lies entirely within the uterus, the external os being of natural size, the diagnosis requires to be very carefully made, as it is easy to mistake a partially inverted uterus for a polypus; still more serious is that error, of which several cases are recorded (I have myself witnessed two), in which a totally inverted uterus has been removed under the belief that it was a vaginal polypus.

The following case, comprising many of the most difficult points, is of interest, as showing that the removal of an intra-uterine polypus may be effected without the delay and trouble required for artificial dilatation of the os :—

M. W., æt 42, a virgin, blanched by continuous uterine hæmorrhage, which had gone on for two months, and increased with the least effort. There had been previous menorrhagia for upwards of a year; the os externum was circular, thin, and distensible, so that the finger could be wormed into the cavity, which was occupied by a polypus distending the internal os, and attached to the fundus by a pedicle of the thickness of the middle finger. I removed the tumour as soon as the patient could be prepared, first incising the os in several directions by means of my hysterotome (p. 186), having so regulated the blades, that only the lower zone of the cervix should be divided. Simple torsion sufficed to free the tumour, which was as large as a hen's egg. The hæmorrhage immediately ceased; the patient recovered without a bad symptom. The incised cervix rapidly healed, and became atrophied.

APLASIA.—The surface of the cervix uteri is sheathed with a pavement epithelium, which is very rapidly removed and renewed. If the balance between these conditions be disturbed, either by increase of the destructive action or any defect in the reparative process, there ensues a denudation, abrasion, or excoriation of the surface, which may occur as a mere ring around the os, or be of such extent as to implicate the whole of the vaginal surface of the cervix. The denuded villi appear rough and raised, and deeper in colour, without that glisten which the healthy mucous surface presents, and feel like velvet to the touch. There is a continuous stillicidium from the raw surface, which becomes yellowish and thick by admixture with the alkaline discharge that proceeds from the interior of the os.

Between this condition and that of true ulceration of the womb there is a wide distinction, and the treatment is proportionably different. In the one case there is simple defect of reparation, in the other there is an active destructive agency. In the former it is only necessary to remove the local cause by which the balance of nutrition has been disturbed, in order to insure renewal of the healthy surface, as commonly seen in extreme cases of prolapsus, where the abrasion round the os immediately heals on restoration of place. In true ulceration the determining cause of the destructive influence (usually constitutional) has to be sought for and removed before the sore be soundly treated. Simple abrasion, or "granular erosion," is of very frequent occurrence; and it is by no means rare to find that the patient has previously suffered from similar symptoms, and recovered without any local treatment. True ulceration of the womb is very seldom met with.

I am led to believe that the majority of cases of erosion of the cervix are either of mechanical origin, or continue because this cause serves to perpetuate some local irritation. Mere digital examination often teaches more than the speculum reveals. Thus the presence of scybalæ in the rectum is at once recognised by the touch: against these hard bodies the delicate tissue of the cervix is impinged by each movement, especially if the patient laces tightly, or has to lift heavy weights, if the uterus be anteverted, or so hypertrophied that the effort of defecation causes it to be forced downwards into the pelvis. Mobility, size, and position are best ascertained by the touch; but the employment of the speculum is essential for correct diagnosis of the state of the surface of the cervix, and to insure that the condition of granular erosion may be duly discriminated. For "this state has been considered one of superficial ulceration; but epithelial abrasion is the only morbid change which exists in cases of this kind, and it is nothing like that which is considered ulceration in other parts of the body. If this were to be considered genuine ulceration we must apply the same term to the simple loss of epidermis after the application of a blister to the skin."*

I have carefully noted the conditions, the treatment, and the result in a very large number of cases, and my opinion very precisely coincides with that expressed by Dr. Tyler Smith.

The local symptoms agree in character with those common to every aplasia which affects the cervix, whether simple granular erosion, true ulceration, aphthous and pustular eruption, or malignant disease; but vary widely in their intensity. There is some vaginal discharge, usually yellowish, and stiffening the linen; but occasionally streaked with blood. There is pain on defecation, especially if costive, as though some sore place were pressed; and there is almost constantly much suffering in the back, chiefly referred to the coccyx, and often described as a bruised feeling, such as would ensue from suddenly sitting down on a hard projection. This very frequent symptom is evidently a reflected sensation, corresponding with that pain of the right shoulder so common in hepatic disorder, and its anatomical explanation is equally precise. About one half of the fourth sacral nerve goes to supply branches to the pelvic viscera and muscles, and sends down a communicating filament to the fifth nerve, which, having emerged at the junction of the sacrum and first coccygeal vertebroid, descends upon the coccygeus muscle, then turns backwards, and ends in the integument on the posterior aspect of the bone.

---

* Dr. Tyler Smith "On Leucorrhœa," p. 82.

These symptoms are notably increased by any local disturbing cause, by strain or effort, by sudden jerks, by prolonged constipation, by overfilling of the bladder, and especially by intercourse, which is frequently followed by bleeding. When commencing the treatment, it is necessary to order that these sources of local irritation be avoided until the trouble is removed.

The speculum must be used in the diagnosis of these affections and to ascertain the progress made. It is rarely required for the purpose of treatment, except in long-neglected cases, where time is saved by insuring at the outset a new and healthy action. In ordinary cases of granular erosion, I believe that the application of solid lunar caustic is not only unnecessary but sometimes prejudicial: I was led to prefer solutions of silver of various strengths from a series of observations made six years ago, and have used them ever since in preference to the caustic point, and with excellent practical result. The solid salt necessarily exercises but a very limited influence, for its caustic or cathæretic action extends only to the parts it touches, on which is soon produced an insoluble and inenergetic film. This consists of chloride of silver, and of that undetermined compound which the salt forms with albumen. Whatever the principles guiding its application (and there can be no doubt of its value in some cases), they differ widely from those which led Higginbotham to advocate its use. He laid especial stress on the endurance of the eschar, which in uterine cases is of course very rapidly loosened and removed. There may be some slight degree of interstitial absorption in that period which elapses before the soluble nitrate is converted into the insoluble chloride.

It was by accident that the solution which I now constantly employ was first brought under my notice. In treating a severe case of granular erosion, I chanced to upset the silver solution (half a drachm to an ounce) previously used. On the emergency I resorted to another preparation of about the same strength, but which had been laid aside as no longer available for its original purpose. It was, in fact, an old photographic nitrate bath, still bright and clear, but which had been so long worked that it had become saturated with iodide of silver and contained a considerable amount of ether. The beneficial effects were so marked when next I saw the patient, that I continued its use, and have employed it largely in similar affections with notable advantage. The rationale of its action may be thus explained: A reparative process is a healthy process; but one requiring local determination for the supply of new material. This is effected in a roundabout way when an eschar is produced by application of caustic to an indolent sore. The textural destruction leads to an energetic determination of blood for repairing the damage, and the original local sore is healed by inducing that same reparative process through which the integrity of tissue is insured during health. A fluid application is absorbed into the tissues just where the special action has to be exercised. This is peculiarly the case where the so-

260 UTERINE DISORDERS.

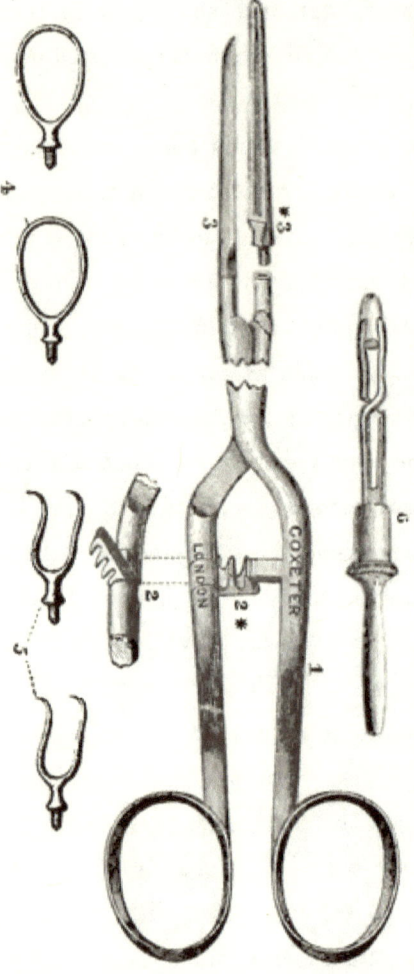

Near the loop-handles, 1 is a ratchet catch, 2*, so that the blades can be firmly locked; this catch is so contrived that it can be freed at will by turning the indented tongue, as seen in fig. 2. The blades (3-3*) firmly grasp the caustic holder (6) if it be required to apply the nitrate. These blades unscrew (3*), and may be replaced by two polypus loops (4), or two vulsellum hooks (5), or one of each may be used.

lution above-mentioned is used, since the ether serves to stimulate capillary absorption.

In those very chronic cases where the bared villi of the cervix almost resemble exuberant granulation, the iodide of silver is especially valuable. To a little of a solution of silver, (a drachm to an ounce), is added a few drops of tincture of iodine, and the flaky whitish deposit which is energetically developed is taken up on a dossil of wool and quickly applied; the speculum being immediately withdrawn, for light acts as a reducing agent. This form of granular erosion is not unfrequent where the uterus is large and soft, and its structure in that unhealthy enfeebled state already described (p. 148).

It is sometimes referred to as the fungous ulcer. In the treatment of granular erosion it is seldom necessary to confine the patient to her bed, but every possible precaution should be enjoined to insure that the cervix be left at rest, in order that it may have opportunity to heal. The dress must be loose, the bladder and bowels relieved without strain, the douche used each day to clear off any accumulated discharge, and a slight astringent lotion injected after its employment, using a suppository at night. Those of lead, of morphia, and of tannin (in the Brit. Pharm.), are among the most useful. In employing the speculum, it is very important to thoroughly clear away all clinging discharge before making any local application. For this purpose, and to subserve a number of other uses, I contrived the "speculum forceps" shown on opposite page.*

Sir J. Y. Simpson directed attention to the occasional occurrence on the cervix of various eruptions, "the vascular, pustular, tubercular, and erythematous orders of Willan and Bateman." In these rare cases it is important to remember that concurrent congestion of the cervix may lead to granular erosion between the eruptive spots, and that these may be greatly modified by the physical conditions of the part. Thus, the scattered pustules sometimes seen on the cervix (and which so strongly resemble acne of the face), may simply result from irritation of an herpetic bleb. They give exit to a drop of pus on being touched with a knife, and the application of the caustic point usually ensures a cure.

---

* Made by Coxeter, Grafton-street East.

A condition closely resembling aphtha of the mouth is occasionally met with; the cervix having on its surface three or four irregular shaped whitish patches with a reddened base. The cases I have seen of this cervical muguet have all occurred in feeble women, whose usual health was much below par— the local application of iodine, and internal administration of aperients with chlorate of potass and bark, succeeded in seven cases where I was able to trace the result. In each there was a large accumulation of retained fæces in the lower bowel. These cases have been erroneously described as diphtheria of the cervix uteri. The application of any strong caustic to the surface is quite inadmissible, and may produce serious mischief.

There is a form of cervical aplasia where the raw surface has a worm-eaten look; with a general resemblance to the condition described as granular erosion, but dotted with a number of minute fossæ, from which there issues a transparent secretion, so abundant that it may stand in beads on the surface of the sore. I conceive that these cases (of which I have carefully observed ten), are examples of herpetic disease of the cervix, chiefly of interest because of their intractability by local applications. In six of these cases a great variety of plans had been tried, in order to effect a cure by topical means. The administration of arsenic proved uniformly successful in my later cases, the sore healing soundly so soon as the medicine began to tell on the system. But even when healed, there remains in these cases, often for many months, a mottled appearance of the cervix; the spots of the original eruption showing with a red hue through the restored superficial membrane.

Of primary syphilitic chancre of the cervix (independent of external ulcer) I have never seen an instance. M. Gibert detected granular erosion in one-third of five hundred venereal cases observed at the Lourcine; but in upwards of three-fourths of these cases there was coincident disease in other parts. Allusion has already been made (p. 236) to certain cases where the presence of a slight syphilitic taint, insufficient to engender the disease, appears to exercise specific influence on the cervix, in modifying the character and retarding the healing of an ordinary erosion. Close observation in a large number of cases has led me to believe that there is one appearance occasionally presented by intractable sores of the cervix which should always lead to further inquiries. This special character is an appearance as of radiating lines, from the os to the circumference of the sore, produced by shallow linear depressions. I think that the persistence of the poison in the system of the husband, if only to that slight extent which is denoted by occasional skin-eruptions, is sufficient to impress this unhealthy character on a pre-existing granular sore of the cervix.

Intractable by local treatment (healing and again recurring with great persistence), these sores rapidly get well whenever the systemic influence of a mercurial alterative is thoroughly established. The formula on page 249 is that which I have found most useful. The great advantage derived, and the absolute immunity which ensued when once the sore was healed, almost induced me to suspect that the mercurial treatment continued to exercise a protective influence. This is not so: just as long as the cervical mucous membrane remains sound, constitutional disease in the male induces no such injurious local effects as ensue when a raw surface is exposed to the contaminating influence. The observances necessary for guarding against any breach of continuity in this mucous membrane have been already described.

True ulceration of the cervix uteri, where there is active destruction of tissue, most commonly accompanies some primary syphilitic disease of the external organs, but there may be found a red and angry sore, the margin being irregular and, as it were, eaten out, where there is no evidence of venereal taint. Such cases are very rare, and I believe always denote that there has been previous granular erosion. This irritable sore of the cervix may, under certain unhealthy conditions, take on a diseased action, in some degree resembling that occurring in superficial indolent sores, and denominated the sloughing ulcer or phagedæna. Application of acid nitrate of mercury to the part, and a pad of oiled wool to prevent mechanical irritation, the thorough evacuation of the bowels, and administration of large doses of opium, will suffice to arrest the progress of the disease and to alleviate the severe suffering. I have seen only three cases of this form of disease; but in each of these was a well-marked strumous taint. Whether this was causative or coincident I do not know. The most marked and frequent cases of true ulceration of the cervix are those in which its character indicates that disease of malignant type has invaded the uterine structure. As the extension of the disease is assuredly fatal, and the evidence as to the value of prompt and decided local treatment in cases of epithelioma and lupus is certainly favourable, it is important to lose no time in adopting the treatment already described, when once the diagnosis has been satisfactorily made out.

INDEX.

ABSCESS, pelvic, 88
Aëtius, his work, 9
Alexandria, school of, 6—13
Amenorrhœa, 112; systemic, 114; ovarian, 118; uterine, 121; treatment of, 115, 118, 119, 122
Ammonia, hydrochlorate of, 59
Ante-curvature of uterus, 64
Anteflexion, 63
Anteversion, 66
Aphtha of cervix, 262
Aplasia, 213, 255
Arabian school, 13—20
Arsenic, use of, 118, 263

BATHS, 12, 93
Blood-poisoning in amenorrhœa, 117

CACOPLASIA, 213, 223
Cancer, 224; treatment of, 229
Cauliflower excrescence, 232
Caustic, use of, 258
Celsus, 7
Change of life, 110
Chlorosis, 112—135

DISLOCATED ovary, 89
Disorders of function, 97—209; place, 43—96; structure, 210—265
Douches, 205
Dysmenorrhœa, 157; systemic, 159; ovarian, 166; uterine, 163; membranous, 186; treatment of, 166, 170, 176, 184

ELECTRICITY in amenorrhœa, 120
Emmenagogues, 113
Epilepsy in women, 161
Epithelial cancer, 232
Ergot in amenorrhœa, 123
Eruptions on cervix, 261

FECUNDITY, natural, 101
Fibrous tumours, 244; treatment of, 249
Flexions, uterine, 63
Function, disorders of, 97

GALVANIC pessaries, 122
Granular erosion, 256; treatment of, 258
Graafian vesicle, 110

HEADACHES in women, 96, 165
Heteroplasiæ, 213, 237
Hydrochlorate of ammonia, use of, 59
Hyperplasia, 213, 238
Hypertrophy, uterine, 238, 242
Hysteria, 198
Hysterotome, its use, 185; new, 186

IGNATIA amara, 116
Inflammation, uterine, 214
Infra-mammary pain, 199
Injections, use of, 12, 94; intra-uterine, 22, 155; per rectum, 177, 231
Intra-uterine pessaries, 83; new spring, 87
Iodide of silver, 259, 260

Iodized cotton, 243
Iron, use of, 116, 156, 201
Irrigateur, 155

JOINT-PAINS in amenorrhœa, 133

LATERAL displacement of uterus, 88
Leeches, use of, 42, 150
Leucorrhœa, 188; definition of, 189; treatment of, 200

MEDICATED suppositories, 10, 261
Menorrhagia, 140; constitutional influence of, 141; periodic, 142; systemic, 144; ovarian, 146; uterine, 147; treatment of, 151
Menstrua alba, 196
Menstrual check, 128
Miscarriage, anteversion causing, 21

NECKAM, Alexander, on menstruation, 98
Neuralgic dysmenorrhœa, 164

OCCLUSION, uterine, 122, 112, 183
Oculus sacerdotum, 99
Order of function, 99; place, 24; structure, 210
Ovarian amenorrhœa, 118; dysmenorrhœa, 166; menorrhagia, 146; sterility, 206
Ovariotomy, 237

PARTHENOGENESIS, 238
Pelvic abscess, 88
Pessaries, air, 14, 82; boxwood and ring, 51; butterfly (Zwancke), 58; Dr. Hodge's, 82; intra-uterine spring (new), 86; medicated (history of), 10; Sir J. Y. Simpson's stem, 84
Pliny on menstruation, 18
Polypus uteri, 250; diagnosis, 252; treatment, 253
Porte caustique, 11
Primerose, Jacobus, 21

Prolapsus, uterine, 48; active, 49; passive, 48; vaginal, 48
Puberty, 107

REST, 93
Retroflexion, 73; cases, 79; causes, 74; pathology, 75; treatment, 76
Retroversion, 73
Rodent ulcer, 233

SOUND, uterine, 12; in diagnosis, 56—67; in treatment. 76; value of, 77
Speculum, use of, 258; history of, 2—19; at Pompeii (B.C. 79), 18; mentioned by Galen (A.D. 200), 6; Aretæus (A.D. 350), 6; Aëtius, (A.D. 500), 10; Paul of Ægina (A.D. 600), 16; Albucasis (A.D. 1350), 16; Rueffus (A.D. 1587), 17; H. Fabricius (A.D. 1620), 16; Gabelchouer (A.D. 1627), 16; Paré (A.D. 1640), 17; Scultetus (A.D. 1650), 14; Wierus (A.D. 1657), 17; Garengeot (A.D. 1727),17; Arnaud (A.D.1728), 17
Split rectus abdominis, 47
Sponge tents, 11, 185
Stays, influence of, 46
Sterility, 205; systemic, 206; ovarian, 206; uterine, 207
Structure, disorders of, 210
Strychnia in amenorrhœa, 116
Suppression of menstruation, 125; from mental influences, 126; from physical causes, 127
Syphilis, 235
Syphilitic sore of cervix, 264

TUBERCLE, 234

ULCERATION of uterus, 221, 255, 264
Urethra, vascular growths in, 240
Uterus, ante-curvature of, 64; anteflexion of, 63; and liver (relations

of), 41; anteversion of, 66; cancer of, 224; development of, 104; epithelioma of, 232; fibrous tumour of, 244; granular erosion of, 256; hypertrophy of, 238—242; injections into, 155; lateral displacement of, 88; occlusion of, 112; 122, 183; prolapsus of, 48, polypus of, 256; retroflexion of, 73; retroversion of, 73; rodent ulcer of, 233; syphilitic implication, 235, 264; ulceration of, 255

VAGINA, as supporting uterus, 32; prolapsus of, 48
Vascular tumours, in urethra, 240; in cervix uteri, 241
Vicarious menstruation, 137

THE END.

www.ingramcontent.com/pod-product-compliance
Lightning Source LLC
Chambersburg PA
CBHW031937230426
43672CB00010B/1954